Every Step of the Way

A Faith Journey Through Breast Cancer

Pam Lillehei

Beaver's Pond Press, Inc.
Edina, Minnesota

Front cover photograph by Tom Lillehei.
The flowers pictured were gifts from friends of the author to encourage her immediately following surgery.

ISBN: 1-890676-71-3

Library of Congress Catalog Card Number: 00-108551

First Printing:
Printed in the United States of America

04 03 02 01 00 6 5 4 3 2

Design and Typesetting By Mori Studio
Edina, MN 55439

This book is dedicated to the memory of
my father and my good friend Valerie
who taught me how to live a joyous life
right up to the very end,
and to all people affected by serious illness.
May you find hope and
encouragement within these pages.

My heartfelt thanks to:
Connie Wilson,
who reviewed this book and
encouraged me to continue writing.

Lyn Ceronsky,
my nurse advisor at the breast cancer center,
who not only reviewed my book but who walked me
through this difficult journey with care and compassion.

My children and ever-patient husband,
who gave me emotional support.
My husband also took care of the technical details
of writing this book. Without his computer skills
I would still be on Chapter One.

My publisher, Milt Adams, who introduced me to everyone
I needed to know to make this book come alive. What a
mentor he has proven to be!

My editor, Connie Anderson, who patiently reviewed my
book and offered excellent advice to make it not only
grammatically correct, but useful to people in crisis.

Mary Ellen Conners, who helped me with the prayer
guidelines and suggestion section, based on her many years
of experience on our church prayer team.

Jack Caravela and Jaana Bykonich at Mori Studio, whose
creativity and sense of style gave the book its artistic design.

Eight very special women who were willing to share
their personal stories of triumph and pain:
Sherry, Kory, Nini, Lois, Julia, Janet, Elaine and Glenda.
I've chosen not to use these women's full names.
They could be your friend, sister, mother,
neighbor or the woman next to you in church,
in line or in your heart. They ranged in age from
mid-40s to mid-70s. Most had children and some were
grandmothers. You will find their thoughts
interspersed into my story.

As we are all aware, not all people are healed.
Since I interviewed these women,
sadly three have died of breast cancer.
Sherry, Elaine and Glenda were praying, faithful,
God-fearing women and yet they died.
I cannot answer the "why."

What I can tell you is that God carried these women
through to the end, granting them and their families
strength and peace. He showed mercy by
sending soft touches and gentle words of comfort,
sometimes from total strangers. I believe physical healing is
secondary. God's love is primary, always there,
in countless ways: a kind deed, a friend's offer to pray,
a meal from a neighbor, a visit from a friend.

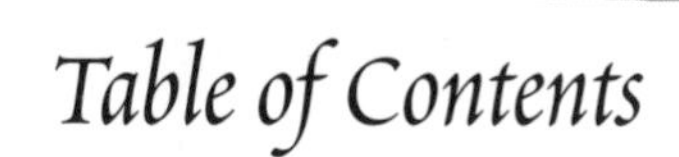

Table of Contents

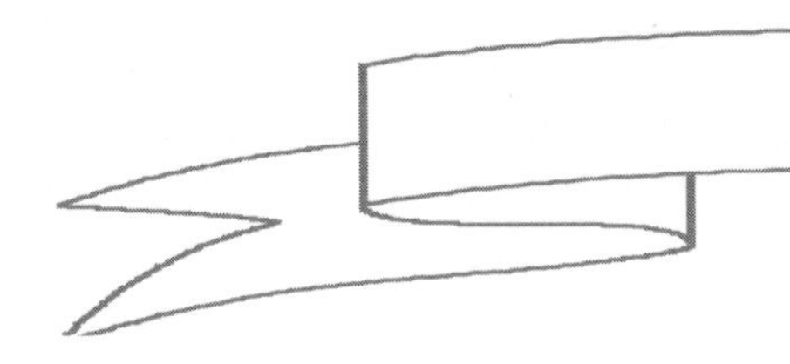

A Message From the Author

This request was printed in our Hope Presbyterian Church newsletter on February 19, 1996.

Share Your Spiritual Journey

Is your breast cancer story full of ways in which God took care of you? When you needed help, or before you were even aware that you were headed for a difficult time, was someone always there to guide you along? My personal experience is full of evidence that God was with me every step of the way, even before I had a diagnosis of breast cancer.

If you have a similar experience you would like to share, I would love to include it in a book I'm writing. The focus will be on how God, by his loving presence, guides and upholds us through breast cancer. Please call or write so our spiritual journeys can be a source of encouragement and hope to others.

Immediately I had three calls. A woman at Hope Presbyterian Church called. Her sister had breast cancer and may want to talk to me. Another woman had just completed her last chemo treatment the day before calling me and she was looking for someone to talk to who would understand how she felt. The third call was from Connie Wilson, a church friend who is also a writer.

Connie said that during her prayer time she had gained insight into her own struggle with procrastination. She explained that it's sometimes difficult to begin a writing project. We agreed to be a source of encouragement to one another, promising to call every Friday to see how our writing was progressing. I viewed Connie's call as God's nudge to get started. This book's completion is due in large part to Connie's patient advice and belief that people would be interested in my faith journey.

Shortly after this newsletter request appeared, I started to get more calls from women who wanted to share their story. I even met two women at a play about breast cancer. After we talked about my book, they too agreed to tell their survivor stories. God brought us together because of the message they had to share. What a joy and privilege it was for me to meet and listen to each woman's faithful and faith journey.

This was how I began writing my book. I have been greatly blessed during trying times. My desire is that you will also be blessed as you read how God demonstrated His love and compassion.

Preface

Every Step of the Way is about my personal experience with breast cancer. I realized early on that God was intervening in very specific ways to ease the sense of fear and panic I felt from the moment I heard the words, "Pam, you have a lump."

As you read my story I hope you can see God's love and grace as He worked out all the minute details of this entire experience. God held my shaking hand and led me, step by step, back to health. When I needed help the most, I received it. Not in a chance occurrence, but instead by God's attendant love for me, a love that was far greater than I had ever realized.

Along with my story I am including similar situations of hope and encouragement from women who voluntarily shared their breast cancer experience with me. My goal is to lessen the fear that most women experience by offering positive examples from women who have fought the fight and did it through God's grace and love.

So, as you read both my account and those of the other women I interviewed, read with a critical eye. Watch for God's constant intervention in very personal ways. I want you to know that the most fearful time of my life became a time of immense peace when I realized what God was doing for me.

He can do the same for you.

Before you start reading my story of faith, I want to share Sherry's story. It says it all—be open to God's demonstrated love and compassion—and the people He may use to show it.

> *My husband John asked me if I was going to church one Sunday. I said, "No, I'm not going to church because I'm mad. I'm not going."*
>
> *On that Sunday morning I was cleaning the barn and it just came to me in my head, "Sherry, if this were your last Sunday on earth, would you want to go to church?" And I said, "Yeah, I'd want to go to church. I like my church. I like the worship service. I love the music. Yeah, I want to go to church."*
>
> *So I went to church. This was summertime, almost the end of June. There weren't many people there. I sat in the pew, near the front, and the whole pew was empty except me. And in comes this woman who comes down and almost sits on my lap, almost on my lap. And my mind is thinking, "Gee, lady, the church is empty. You could sit anywhere. Why here?"*
>
> *Well, I'm in church. I tell myself, "Be nice, Sherry. You know, get these icky thoughts out of your head."*
>
> *And it was a good worship service. At the end of the service we stood to greet each other. This woman who had sat so close to me said, "My name is Lillian." I told her my name. Then she said, "I'm just going to give you a big Christian hug."*
>
> *As she hugged me, she said, "Do you have any prayer requests?"*

And I said, "Well, yes," and I told her my story.

"Praise God! I prayed that He would send me somebody to pray for," Lillian told me.

That was really a demonstration that God is there every step of the way, no matter what! There He was. I didn't know I needed Lillian that morning. I didn't have a clue. But I was obedient. I went to church. And God provided for me. That is a really significant story for me. I've kept in touch with Lillian. She's been a real faithful prayer partner for me since that time. I didn't know her before—not at all.

Sherry

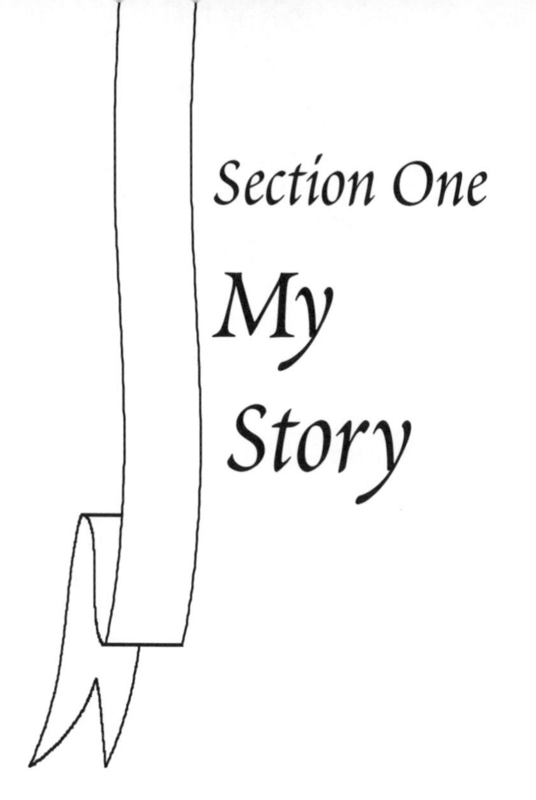

Section One

My Story

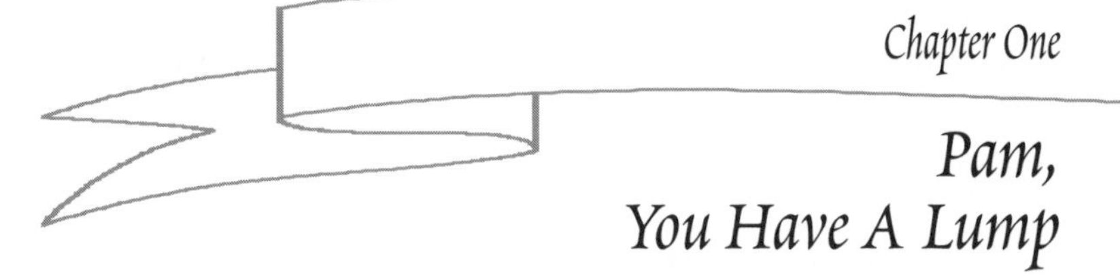

Chapter One

Pam, You Have A Lump

Author's Note: All physicians' names have been changed.

"I need to tell you. My maternal grandmother had breast cancer. Do you really think it's safe for me to be on hormonal therapy?" I explained to my gynecologist.

I was nervous and fearful about my gynecologist's near insistence that I take estrogen. My grandmother's breast cancer was always in the back of my mind. Not as a fearful threat of imminent doom, but as a realization that I could be at an increased risk for breast cancer and should therefore be careful about medications. Consequently, I was reluctant to take my doctor's advice without challenging his reasons.

"Look at the statistics on heart disease and osteoporosis," Dr. Rosen said. You should be more concerned about getting a heart attack or breaking a bone than you are about getting breast cancer. That's the point of taking estrogen—it's helpful in preventing these diseases."

It was a decision only I could make. I knew that. I had undergone a complete hysterectomy that summer. Without ovaries, I knew I was without my natural protection against heart disease and osteoporosis. But with my grandmother's mastectomy clearly on my mind, I needed to be convinced that taking estrogen, as Dr. Rosen wanted me to do, was worth the risk.

"What if I get breast cancer anyway?"

"Studies have shown that the cancer is more localized in women on hormonal treatment than in those who are not," Dr. Rosen explained.

"Well, okay, I'll give it a try," I told him reluctantly, still not certain that I would swallow the pills once I had them.

As I dropped off my prescription, I asked the female pharmacist, "What do you know about estrogen? My doctor thinks I should take this because of a recent complete hysterectomy. But honestly, taking this really frightens me. I'm so glad you're a woman so I can ask you for advice. What would you do if you were in my shoes?"

"From all the reading I've done I would be comfortable taking estrogen when my time comes. I've already made that decision, in fact. I don't see a problem," the pharmacist replied.

This pharmacist's counsel seemed to be a green light to go ahead and take the estrogen. After all, not only was she a woman, she was a professional who I figured knew about these things, had studied the scientific literature and had made an informed decision. I trusted her expertise.

I filled the prescription that day and thus began my time on hormonal therapy. I never actually gave it a second thought. Taking that medication became routine, in fact so routine that I was irritated when in October, about a year later, the pharmacist handed me a smaller refill bottle. He explained, "You'll have to see your gynecologist, Dr. Ferguson. (I had changed to a female gynecologist. I felt she was more patient and understanding of a woman's needs.) She won't authorize any more than a one-month supply. I'm sorry, I know you've been getting a three-month supply, but those are the rules. She told us very clearly, 'No exam, no medication.'"

Irritated at what to me was an inconvenience and something I thought was unnecessary, I made an appointment to see Dr. Ferguson on November 11.

Don't get me wrong. I liked Dr. Ferguson. She was in her mid-thirties, the mother of three, calm, easy-going, always comfortably attired in a long, casual cotton print dress with her white doctor's coat hanging loosely from her shoulders. She had a neat and orderly suburban office, a large friendly staff, and a down-home appeal that made me feel like I was chatting with my best friend.

As I sat on the examining table clad in the customary paper gown, she glanced at my chart, then turned to look me straight in the eye. "What can I do for you today, Pam?"

"I'm here because I have to be, Dr. Ferguson. No offense to you or anything, but I hadn't intended to see you for another year. I thought patients who had had a hysterectomy didn't need a yearly pap. I was going to save you and me the time by waiting a year. But the pharmacist told me you wouldn't renew my estrogen prescription without a visit to you, so here I am."

"That's right. We think it's necessary to see patients once a year when they're on estrogen," the doctor replied.

"By the way, I had a mammogram a couple weeks ago. Did you get the results?" I asked.

"Yes. In fact I remember your report distinctly. I read the results just yesterday in my downtown office and they were normal. Completely normal."

I was relieved. Ever since I could remember, I was having regular mammograms because of my grandmother's breast cancer. I scheduled these on my own and always at the same clinic so they'd be sure to notice any changes from exam to exam. I guess I'm good for another year, I thought to myself.

"Pam, lie down and I'll examine you." She examined my right breast first, her fingers making the customary circular route around the breast, carefully feeling for any abnormalities. She did the same careful search on the left breast.

"Do you examine your breasts every month?" she asked as she reexamined my right breast.

"No, because my breasts are so lumpy. Fibrocystic I believe you call it. Anyway, I wouldn't know a good lump from a bad one. I just need an expert like you to tell me what's normal. I'm relying on you, Doctor."

"Well," she said, "the right breast feels different from the left. There seems to be a small lump. Here. Can you feel this?"

She placed my hand on the outer edge of my right breast. Sure enough, a lump!

My heart fell. This was a lump. A breast lump. How did it get there? What did this mean? Wasn't my mammogram negative?

Dr. Ferguson told me to relax. She explained that most lumps are benign. An easy way to prove it would be for her to do an immediate needle biopsy. "All I need to do is insert this needle into your breast lump, draw out some fluid, and then have the fluid analyzed. It's a very quick and easy procedure," she explained.

As I laid there, I remembered that years ago I had been more cautious and worried about breast cancer. I had even visited a breast clinic where I had talked to a nurse and had watched a video on breast care and self-examination. At the conclusion of my visit, that nurse had given me a prosthetic breast and had asked me to find the hidden lump inside. Upon reflection, that prosthetic lump that I had so easily found years ago felt just like the one I could now feel in my own breast.

What was happening to me? This was supposed to be a quick visit. Just a casual dropping in for a routine exam so I could get another year's go-ahead for estrogen and then I was to be merrily on my way. Life as usual.

Not so! As I stared at the ceiling, waiting for Dr. Ferguson to get her needle ready, I felt a lump begin to form in my throat. I swallowed hard and tried to fight back tears. "Oh, please, God, don't let me cry yet. I want to do that alone. Not here."

After two attempts Dr. Ferguson explained, "I can't seem to withdraw any fluid. You'll need to have this checked out in the next week or two. I don't think it's urgent, but I do believe you should have it looked at. Your primary care doctor can refer you to a surgeon for a biopsy."

"Do you do biopsies here?" I asked anxiously. I had hoped she could perform the biopsy right then and there. I wanted to know what this lump was. It may not have been urgent to her, but to me it was critical that I find out what I was facing, and the sooner the better.

She kindly explained that her practice only does obstetrical and gynecological surgeries.

Disappointed, I got dressed in a daze. The next thing I recall I was sitting on a chair outside Dr. Ferguson's examining room, waiting for the results of a routine blood test. I was oblivious to the doctors, nurses and patients who came and went around me, and I didn't really care about the blood test, compared to the unknown I now faced.

I felt so alone and disconnected from the rest of the world. All I could think of was that nasty breast lump and the urgency I felt to get it diagnosed. My world had become one dimensional. I had a lump and I wanted it removed immediately! Nothing else mattered.

It was 3:30 Friday afternoon when I finally left her office. Although I wanted to cry, and expected that I would do so as soon as I left her office, I managed to walk briskly to the parking lot without a tear in my eyes. I unlocked my car door, sat tensely erect behind the steering wheel, tightly pursed my lips, and focused my thoughts on getting to my suburban clinic. I told myself that if I concentrated on the drive and not on the bad news I had just received, I would be able to see a doctor immediately so I could get my surgical referral. Even though I remembered Dr. Ferguson telling me I didn't need to get a biopsy right away, I was so anxious and terrified that was all I could think about.

The drive wasn't bad. I had expected to cry all the way to the clinic, but I managed to hold it all in. I don't know how, except that I was so focused on my goal that I just kept telling myself, "Get there. Get there, first. Don't fall apart yet. Do that later. You have to focus now. Focus, Pam. Focus."

I prayed as I drove, "Please, God, help me. You know the panic I am feeling right now. I have a lump, God. A lump! You've got to help me. I'm afraid that if I walk into that clinic and someone doesn't treat me kindly, I won't even be able to tell them what I need. And you know what I need and you know the bureaucracy that faces me. I can't even go to a surgeon on my own. I have to see my primary care doctor first. I'm worried about time here, God. This is only the first step. I'm afraid, God. Please, make sure I can talk to someone at the clinic with an understanding and compassionate heart. Don't let me meet someone who's had a bad day because I am fragile right now. I need loving care to protect me, God. Compassion, God. I need compassion."

At 4 p.m. I pulled into the clinic parking lot. I had managed to drive about 20 miles without a tear. I congratulated myself.

I rushed into the clinic and explained to the woman at the counter that I needed to see a doctor right away for a surgical referral. "All the doctors have left for the day," she explained, "but you can make an appointment for Monday. Please spell your last name for me."

I couldn't believe it. Here I had driven so purposefully, so controlled, only to be told there was no one for me to see that day. No doctor. I had a lump and there was no doctor for me to tell. No doctor.

I began to spell my name, "L-I-L-L." I stopped. I could no longer speak. What was wrong with me? All I needed to do was tell her my name, get my appointment and leave.

But it wasn't that simple. Telling someone that I had a lump, verbalizing what was going on with me was more difficult than I had imagined. It had been easy to stay focused and hold back the tears as I drove to the clinic, but once I had to open my mouth and tell another human being that I had a problem, it made my situation all too real. Fear and desperation were beginning to take hold. Tears flooded my cheeks as I tried to finish spelling my name.

Once I was able to calm down and get my appointment made, I thanked this kind woman for being so patient and understanding with me. As I was about to walk out of the clinic door, thankful that God had answered my prayer, she added, "I'm a breast cancer survivor. Here's my card. I'm Barb. Call me any time you need to talk."

"Wait a minute," I thought. Who said anything about breast cancer? I had a benign lump. Why did Barb mention the "C" word? I did not expect to need any further conversation with Barb. It crossed my mind to wonder what God was up to, but I quickly dismissed the thought.

When I had my surgery, a nurse came up to me right in that holding room before you have surgery. And she whispered in my ear, "I had the same surgery a few years ago and I'm going to visit you." And she did. And I thought that was so nice because that was real hopeful since I didn't know anyone who had breast cancer or who had had surgery or anything. God plants people where you need them.

Nini

Chapter Two

The Retreat

About a month before the lump was found, my friend Kory had suggested that we sign up for the women's retreat on November 12 and 13, sponsored by our Sunday School class. "I don't really want to go, Kory, but if you're looking for someone to be there with you, then okay, I'll go with you," I told her.

I don't know why I hesitated. What woman wouldn't want to get away for a day and a half of peace and quiet? But, without Kory's prodding, I know I would have stayed home and missed the blessing that God had waiting for me.

The retreat was held in an idyllic setting just south of the Twin Cities. There was a cozy lodge with a fireplace, comfortable couches for long chats, and a huge picture window overlooking beautifully wooded acres. There was a pool, hot tub and sauna, walking paths through the woods, a small pond with some wildlife, a common dining hall and a small chapel.

The theme for the weekend was "Encouragement." A pastoral intern from our church began her presentation by defining the word *encourage*: "To inspire with courage, spirit, or hope; to spur on; to give hope or promise; to comfort."

She went on to explain that encouragement comes in many different ways. When she mentioned that God uses other people to give us hope and encouragement, I felt compelled to share my story with the group.

"I have to tell all of you what happened to me yesterday. God encouraged me! He answered my prayer and sent me a woman who offered me comfort. What you're saying is true. I have proof."

I then got up out of my chair, walked up beside the speaker and stood in front of thirty women and shared my very personal story. I began with Dr. Ferguson's discovery of the lump, to the ineffectiveness of the needle biopsy, to my tearless but fearful drive to the clinic. I told them that my grandmother had had breast cancer, so the thought that this could be happening to me had crossed my mind. Then I explained to them how I met Barb, a total stranger, who offered to comfort me, to give me hope. By the time I finished sharing, many of us were in tears.

As part of this retreat we were given a worksheet and about an hour in which to study and pray alone. We could go anywhere on the grounds. I chose to sit at a table in front of the large picture window that overlooked the barren trees of fall, now covered by a fresh noon snowfall.

The worksheet began with these words: "It's actually quite amazing to think that this God of ours, who has a universe to run, takes the time to encourage and comfort us. The following verses give some reasons why God does so."

The verses that meant the most to me were:

Praise be to the God and
Father of our Lord Jesus Christ,

the Father of compassion and
the God of all comfort,

who comforts us in all our troubles,
so that we can comfort those
in any trouble with the comfort
we ourselves have received from God.

For just as the sufferings of Christ
flow over into our lives,
so also through Christ
our comfort overflows.

II CORINTHIANS 1:3-5

These verses told me that I would not be alone and that in the midst of my trouble and uncertainty about my medical condition I could hold onto the faithfulness of God. He had already demonstrated His compassion by answering my very first prayer for help when He provided Barb as an earthly comforter. This gave me a sense of assurance that He would not abandon me down the road.

After completing the worksheet, I decided to get up and stretch for a while and look for the nearest restroom. I left my table and walked past several other women who were studying in the same room. Then I wandered out into the hall. Before I could find a restroom, I came upon a chapel across the hall. The door was closed but I felt a tug at my heart to go inside. As I opened the door I discovered a very tiny room, but complete with an altar, a railing and kneeling space and two short rows of chairs.

I sat down in the back row, behind Marilyn, another retreat attendee. As I sat there in silence, my heart told me that the best thing to do at that moment would be to kneel at the altar and pray about my fear and anxiety. I needed to tell God what was going on and how worried I was.

The altar has always been an important place for me. It was where I had accepted Christ as a young adult and it was where I brought my fears when I was pregnant with our daughter Kyrsten and fearful of having a third miscarriage. There I had prayed for strength and health and the blessing of a new birth.

Just as I was thinking how I wanted to go up to this little altar, Marilyn turned around and said, "Do you want to go to the altar to pray?"

I took one look at her, and with tears in my eyes, simply nodded. I was overwhelmed at the simultaneous timing of her question and my desire to kneel at that tiny altar.

As we knelt there together, we held hands as she prayed for me, "Father, heal Pam. May this lump in her breast be benign."

At that time I was expecting the worst, and the thought of asking God for the lump to be benign had never occurred to me. I was glad Marilyn prayed this prayer and I certainly hoped God would honor her request.

Tears continued to roll down my cheeks as I realized that God was there in that tiny chapel. He had placed Marilyn in that first row chair to tend to my needs. She comforted and blessed me and as she prayed the prayer I couldn't even think to pray, my uneasy spirit was quieted.

The entire retreat experience was like that—a time of true sharing where everyone became very open and honest. It was exactly what I needed—a time of preparation for what I was about to face.

> *I told my two closest neighbors, "You were like the love of God to me when I couldn't pray. You said the prayers I couldn't say. You represented all of that to me that I couldn't do myself. I want you to know that you were God's instrument in my life."*
>
> **Julia**

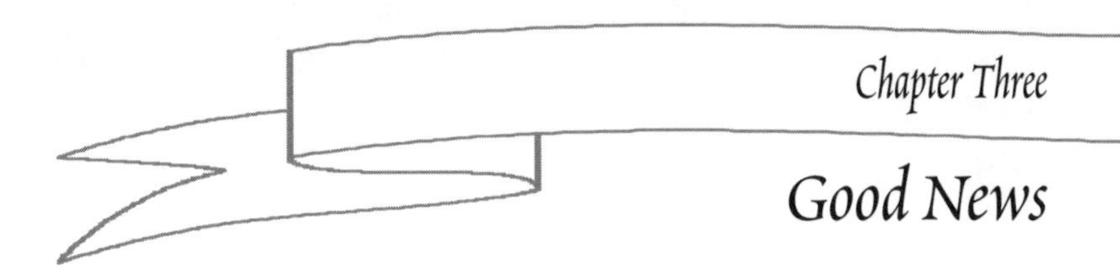

Chapter Three

Good News

On Monday, November 14, I was back at the clinic, this time with an appointment to see my primary care doctor.

"Dr. Samuelson," I began, "you've got to help me. I have a breast lump and I need to see a surgeon today. I've been worrying about this since last Friday when my gynecologist found it. All you need to do is give me the referral and I'll be gone."

"I can understand your sense of urgency, but the usual procedure is to do an ultrasound of the lump first because the surgeon likes to see those pictures before performing a biopsy," he explained.

I couldn't believe what he was telling me. I faced another roadblock, one more hurdle before I was allowed to see a surgeon. Why was this procedure taking so long?

"We can do the ultrasound in this clinic and then you'll be all set. I guess I should ask you, first of all, do you have a surgeon?"

"No. I used to, but he retired. Can you recommend a good one?"

"I sure can. I wholeheartedly recommend Dr. Hill. He has performed surgery on my dad. He's excellent! I wouldn't let just anybody operate on my dad, you know."

"Sounds fine with me. Where do we go from here?" I asked impatiently.

Dr. Samuelson's nurse worked out the details. I was to see the ultrasound technician the next morning and then go to see Dr. Hill in the afternoon.

The next day I showed up at the clinic for the ultrasound.

A perky young technician came into the examining room. "Just lie down and relax," she said. "This is easy and painless." She squeezed some jelly-like substance on my right breast and then moved her wand-type instrument over it, searching for the lump that I had pointed out to her.

"Oh, here it is!" she exclaimed as she showed me on the screen. "This is nothing. Certainly nothing to worry about. Look, see for yourself."

"Really?" I said, surprised and relieved. "What do you think the surgeon will do?" I questioned.

"The surgeon will do absolutely nothing," she assured me. "Why, if they biopsied every lump in a woman's breast, women would be full of holes!"

"What good news! You've certainly made my day!" I thanked her as she gave me the ultrasound pictures to take to Dr. Hill.

All this worry had been for nothing. Maybe I wouldn't even need a biopsy. What relief.

Chapter Four

Bad News

Once I was re-diagnosed with breast cancer, I really can't explain how important prayer became in my life. The fact that I knew other people were praying for me made such a difference. I feel that I am where I am in my recovery today because of prayer. I started believing in the power of prayer. In my Christmas letter I asked people to pray for me because I had breast cancer. When I got cards back from people they told me they had me in their prayers. Then I heard from my husband's relative who put me on her prayer chain at her church. That really, really did something to me. Knowing that a whole congregation was praying for me. I also learned that a group of friends all prayed for me at the same time. I thought this was real special.

Lois

I walked into Dr. Hill's St. Paul surgical clinic. The tiny waiting room was overflowing. Patients and family members sat in every chair; some even waited in the hallway. How could there be so many people needing a surgeon?

I felt so sorry for all these people. One couple, I supposed to be in their sixties, sat in silence, looking at each other with big sad eyes. I wondered if she had breast cancer. I imagined all kinds of unhappy stories.

I thanked God I was just there to have Dr. Hill confirm that the ultrasound pictures I was holding did indeed show a benign lump.

The nurse called my name and I was taken down a narrow hall to a small examining room.

Dr. Hill, a tall handsome man about my age, as I later discovered, welcomed me with a big hello and a handshake.

"So, you're here about a lump?" he questioned. "Let's get some of your family history before I examine you."

I began by telling him about my grandmother's breast cancer. I went on to explain how my lump had been discovered by my gynecologist but that I had proof with me, from the ultrasound technician, that my lump was nothing to worry about.

"Yes, most lumps are benign. Why don't you get undressed and I'll be back in to take a look."

Once again I found myself on an examining table, only this time, I was the one pointing out the lump to the doctor. "Dr. Hill, what do you think this is?" I asked as I showed him the lump in my breast.

After careful examination he said in a reassuring tone, "I'm 95 percent sure this is benign, Pam. But," he continued, "I take an aggressive approach. I don't watch lumps. I believe that's risky. I recommend that you have it biopsied. I'm currently treating a woman who had been advised by another doctor to just watch her lump. She is now in big trouble—the cancer has metastasized. Her outlook is grim. I don't want to take this chance with you."

That couple in the waiting room, I thought. I imagined she was the one he was talking about. No wonder they looked so sad.

"What about the ultrasound pictures I brought you? Can't you just look at those?" I asked.

"No. Those are only useful to me if I'm looking at them while they're being done. The still pictures don't show me what I need to see."

I was puzzled. Dr. Samuelson had said I needed these pictures. The technician had told me my lump was nothing based on what she had seen, but Dr. Hill wouldn't even look at them. I felt as if had wasted precious time.

I did however feel good about Dr. Hill's tentative diagnosis that my lump was benign. I decided to think positively as I awaited my upcoming biopsy scheduled for the following Monday, November 21.

That Sunday my husband Tom and I attended our adult Sunday School class. At the beginning of the class a prayer was said for me and the breast biopsy I was going to have the following day. It felt good to have the class pray out loud for me and ask for God's protection. It took some of the weight off my shoulders.

The guest teacher that day told the class that his wife Karen had had cancer and chemotherapy which meant certain adjustments for their family. He didn't mention what kind of cancer she had dealt with, but made it sound like it had been pretty serious.

After class, Karen approached me. "Are you Pam?" she questioned. When I nodded she said, "I am a breast cancer survivor. I would be glad to help you in any way I can. Please don't hesitate to call."

I thanked her for her kindness, but at the time was confident that I would not need to talk to her. My lump was benign.

Although I believed I wasn't going to need Karen or anyone like her, at the same time I was puzzled why God would send these two particular women—Barb from the clinic and now Karen—to tell me they had survived breast cancer. Up until I talked to those total strangers, I was naturally worried that my lump might be malignant. But until I had the biopsy to prove otherwise, I remained cautiously optimistic and hopeful that I would not end up with breast cancer. After all, Marilyn had prayed for my lump to be benign, the ultrasound technician was sure it was nothing, and now, even Dr. Hill said he was 95 percent sure I had nothing to fear.

By Monday morning, however, the day of the biopsy, my mood had changed. I couldn't get my mind off Barb and Karen. I feared that it was no coincidence that I had met them.

As we stood in our bedroom that morning, preparing to leave for the hospital, I reached out to Tom and said in a faint voice, "I need a big hug."

As he put his arms around me and tried to swallow me up in his love, I confessed that I was scared. "Oh, Tom, hold me tight. I'm afraid God has been trying to give me a warning about what I am soon to find out. I've now had two cancer survivors come up to me to offer help. I'm convinced these women were sent by God with a message for me. And I'm afraid the message is that I have breast cancer!"

I put my head on his shoulder and wept quietly. I felt numb.

He gave me a big reassuring squeeze. As he wiped the tears from my cheeks and stroked my head, he tried his best to calm my fears. "I don't think you have cancer, Pam. God has given you these women as helpers, just in case you need them. Don't worry. You're going to be just fine."

We checked into the hospital for the biopsy. I was given a type of anesthesia that kept me awake but not real alert, plus Novocain to deaden the biopsy area.

As I lay on the operating table, awake but groggy from the anesthetic, Dr. Hill began cutting away the lump. He and the nurses chatted about the music playing in the background and I was glad to join in. Why had I been so fearful in the morning when I told my husband I needed a hug? Tom was right. Everything was going to be fine.

As the surgery progressed, however, I noticed a subtle change in the once carefree banter. No more lighthearted conversations about music. And as Dr. Hill kept cutting, I was beginning to hurt. "More anesthetic, Doctor," the nurse advised. "Pam is grimacing."

Dr. Hill completed the surgical procedure. "I'm not quite sure what the status of your lump is at this point," he said. "It does not look as I had expected before the surgery, but we'll wait for the lab results. You relax and I'll be in to talk to you shortly."

I was wheeled into the post-op waiting room where my husband joined me. As I nibbled some toast and sipped hot tea, I told Tom that Dr. Hill seemed to cut out more than he had anticipated and that he was no longer so convinced that the lump was benign.

In about half an hour, Dr. Hill walked somberly into my recovery room and immediately sat down in the chair to my left. I could tell by his downcast eyes and his careful selection of words that the news was not good. "I wish I didn't have to tell you this, Pam, but you have breast cancer. I'm so sorry. This was totally unexpected."

Although the words were a shock to hear, they came as no surprise. Part of me had been prepared by the two women God had sent. They had been sent to ease the burden, and in a sense, by their very presence and healthful appearance, to tell me that they had survived and so would I.

> *When the surgeon came back in after my biopsy and told me that I did indeed have a malignancy, I was so angry at God that day. I remember going to the restroom and literally shaking my fist in the air at God. "I hate you! I hate you! Why did you let this happen?"*
>
> **Julia**

Chapter Five

What Will I Look Like?

I took a little prosthetic kit to my doctor that I thought he could show to women to make it easier for them after surgery. I thought that would be a nice little way that I could have helped someone without ever really knowing. It doesn't really matter that I wouldn't know. The important thing is to help others.

Julia

Dr. Hill tried to soften the blow. He told me the pathologist would be running more tests, but they were both sure it was malignant. "We can discuss options later, Pam, after you've had a while to digest everything that has just happened," he said.

"Dr. Hill," I began, "I've always known what I would do if I were in this situation. I want a mastectomy. In fact, I might even want you to take the other breast, too."

I doubt that he had many women give him an immediate decision like this, but for me it was easy. I had grown up with my grandmother's example. To her, a mastectomy was no big deal, and it wouldn't be a big deal for me either. And, if I were going to have one breast removed, why not have both taken off at the same time?

Dr. Hill went on to explain that I did have another option—a lumpectomy (where the cancerous lump and some surrounding tissue are removed), followed by six weeks of radiation. He said research seemed to indicate survival rates were comparable to a mastectomy.

"That's fine to know, but I just wouldn't feel like the lumpectomy would be right for me. I'd rather go for the treatment that's been around for a long time. How soon can we schedule surgery? Is this Friday okay?"

I was in a hurry to get the surgery behind me. Now that I knew what needed to be done, I wanted it done, and done now!

"I'm going to be gone on Friday. That's the day after Thanksgiving. The soonest I could operate would be Monday. How's that?"

"Sounds good to me. It's not as soon as I'd like, but that will have to do."

"About removing your other breast as well, I only do one to two of these surgeries per year. I really don't recommend it, but if it's what you want, I'll do it for you. We can talk about that later in the week after you've had more time to think about it."

I left the hospital with a packet of information on the nearby breast center and the name of Lyn, the nurse specialist who worked there. "Give her a call, Pam. She's a great person to talk to. She'll be able to give you lots of information and reading materials on breast cancer. She's an excellent resource for someone in your situation."

On the way home I told Tom that I wanted to stop by my folks' house to tell them the news in person, not over the phone. They were already dealing with my dad's rectal cancer diagnosis six months before.

I walked in the house and looked at my mother and dad, standing side-by-side in the living room. How could I give them one more piece of bad news? "Let's sit down," I suggested. "We've just come from my biopsy. The news is not what we expected. Not what Dr. Hill expected either. I have breast cancer."

My parents sat in silence. They were stunned! They didn't know what to say.

"I need a hug," I said, as I began to cry. I got up off the couch, walked over to my mom and took her hand in mine. She stood up and we wept together, clutching each other in fear. "What's happening to this family?" she asked.

I returned to work the next day and shared the news with my surprised colleagues. (I worked part-time in a school district's administrative offices.) It was not the diagnosis that any of us expected. The superintendent's secretary was very concerned—so concerned, in fact, that she stood in my office and began to cry. As I held her she asked me, "Isn't it supposed to be the other way around? Aren't you supposed to be crying and me comforting you?" A breast cancer diagnosis has rippling affects.

I talked to Dr. Hill that same afternoon to get the pathology report. Since I don't believe in dwelling on the negative, let me just say it was Stage 1—very early cancer. I felt fortunate, indeed. We talked again about him removing the left breast, the one without cancer. I was leaning that way, but as yet hadn't decided. "If that's what you really want, I'll remove the other breast as well. That will be no problem," he reassured me.

I felt confident that Dr. Hill cared about my concerns and was grateful that he would respect my wishes and go with whatever decision I made. I didn't have to justify my reasons to him.

He explained that I would be in the hospital one to two days and come home with drains sticking out of my sides. He told me to discontinue taking estrogen, but he thought it had not caused the cancer. He believed the two major things to deal with would be the psychological aspect of losing the breasts and the numbness under the arm.

Since I was born with only one hand, my right, I was concerned about him cutting the nerves under my right arm. He assured me that only the armpit would be numb. My hand would not be affected because to remove the lymph nodes, only the nerves under the armpit would be cut. Nothing else. Naturally, I was relieved.

On November 23 at 7:11 a.m. I got a call from a close friend from church. This was no ordinary call. He told me that the daughter of a couple in our Bible study had been killed in a car accident the night before—on her way to feed the homeless for Thanksgiving.

"No! I can't believe it! I can't believe it! Oh, no!" I cried. I could no longer talk—tears choked out my words. I had to hang up. I was in shock. I needed to get down on my knees and pray for her and her family.

This young woman's death put my diagnosis of cancer in perspective. My focus quickly shifted from myself to that family. After all, I was not going to die tomorrow from cancer, but she was gone. In an instant. It was so final. No second chance, no hope for survival like I had.

Despite my diagnosis, we celebrated Thanksgiving in grand style. We had 24 people over for dinner. It was great to be busy. I needed to occupy my mind and fill up my time. I didn't want to think too much about what lay ahead. We even experimented with a new dressing—wild rice in combination with the traditional sage and bread stuffing. It was GREAT! Tom and I kept complimenting each other on how delicious it was. My upcoming surgery was only whispered to the women. We weren't letting it be the focus of the day. We had a lot to be thankful for and we were celebrating.

Thanksgiving Friday I awoke with a sense of urgency about my situation. Now I had to face the reality of breast cancer and make some quick decisions. Monday, the day of surgery, was only three days away and I had not even thought about the breast cancer since hearing of that fatal crash. I felt a bit rushed and panicked to decide for sure what I was going to do. Did I really want to have both breasts removed?

My biggest concern that morning was wanting to know what I would look like. I recalled seeing my grandmother's scar when I was a little girl. To me it was not ugly or disfiguring, just a part of my grandmother. Would I look like her I wondered? That wouldn't be bad.

I also wanted to read about breast cancer. I remembered that Dr. Hill had recommended *Dr. Susan Love's Breast Book.* I decided to call Lyn at the breast center, since Dr. Hill had spoken so highly of her. Maybe she could answer some of my questions.

When I called the center I was told it was Lyn's day off. My heart fell. What would I do now?

"I'll page her for you," the secretary offered. "She always answers her page. I'll have her call you."

It wasn't long before Lyn returned my call. I explained, "I'm having surgery on Monday, a double mastectomy, I think. I need to see what I will look like. Do you have any pictures? I'd also like some books to read. This is my day for decision making. I know I should have done all this sooner, but can you help me?"

"I'd be glad to meet you at the breast center. Come on down and we'll see what we can find. I'm sure I have a picture or two I can show you and lots of books I can recommend from our library."

I called my neighbor to see if she would go with me for moral support. My husband would have gone, had I asked him. I just decided I needed a woman with me for this. My neighbor, Lee, said she'd be happy to go with me. Her mother had died of breast cancer years before, so later I questioned whether this had been too painful for her. She didn't seem to mind and I was grateful for her company. I was afraid I would be overcome by fear and sadness and need someone to pick up the pieces.

Lyn was an answer to prayer. She was a kind, patient and gentle person who listened to my questions and gave me more than I had even expected. She had an extensive library with an excellent selection of books related to breast cancer. I checked out several, including Susan Love's book.

Lyn showed me the drainage tube that Dr. Hill had spoken about—a long plastic tube attached to a sort of rubber ball with a plastic pouch. She said this would drain fluid for several days after surgery and that I would have four of them inserted, but probably have some removed before going home.

She also showed me some different kinds of prostheses and a mastectomy bra. Most importantly, however, she had found two books with pictures of real women who had had mastectomies. I was able to look at those pictures and imagine myself without breasts. "Not bad," I told Lyn. "I can live with that." Appearance was not a big issue with me to begin with, but I just had to know ahead of time how bad or how good I was going to look. Now I knew and I felt a sense of peace.

I went home and devoured those books. One particular book which recounted the breast cancer stories of ten women helped me cement my decision to have both breasts removed. Several of these woman ultimately had their second breast removed because of a breast cancer recurrence years later.

That evening, Tom and I decided to go spend some time with the grieving family to offer comfort and support. When we drove up we noticed cars lining both sides of the streets. I wondered aloud if all this was appropriate for the family. The girl's mom assured us that this was exactly what they needed at this time. She was hoping for total exhaustion so that when people left she might be able to sleep and get a reprieve from the awful reality of their daughter's death.

People were wall to wall in the living room. Some I knew; many were new faces. As we sat around and talked about the daughter and the kind of small talk that happens between strangers, I overheard one women talk about the American Cancer Society, mentioning that she was a volunteer. Of course, my ears perked up.

"What do you do for the American Cancer Society?" I inquired.

"I'm a Reach to Recovery volunteer. My name is Ann."

"Oh, Ann, I'm so glad you are here. Could I talk to you? I'm going to have a mastectomy on Monday." I knew that Reach to Recovery volunteers were themselves breast cancer survivors, so I was very excited to meet her.

Ann moved her chair next to mine. For the next two hours she explained her double mastectomy and all the details I would need to know, including how to care for my arms after lymph node removal.

My curiosity centered around all that breast skin. "What will I look like?" I asked. "What do they do with all that breast skin?"

"Would you like to see?" Ann asked.

"Would I! It's something I've wanted to see since I woke up this morning. You are an answer to prayer," I told her.

Ann led me into the bathroom where she showed me her mastectomy scars. They looked very much the way I remembered my grandmother's.

WOW! Not only had God given me a fellow breast cancer survivor to talk to, He had given me a bold, not self-conscious sort who was willing to show me her scars. My desire to know what I would look like had led me from pictures in Lyn's office to a flesh and blood example of God's love and care for every detail of my life.

I was now prepared for Monday's surgery.

> *I had a roommate with a loud, noisy medical machine. I remember hearing that machine. I remember waking up so full of fear, I just cried and cried. I said, "God, you know, if I could just feel a human hand. I'm so lonely and scared. If I could just feel a human hand, I know I'd be okay." Instantly, a nurse came over to my bed, picked up my hand and held it as she asked, "Sherry, are you all right?" And I said, "Wow, I am now!" The reason the noisy machine is so important is because I know no one in the hall heard me muttering or crying or anything because no one could hear a thing over that machine. I never saw that nurse again. I think that was an angel, and if not an angel, God's instant answer to prayer.*
>
> **Sherry**

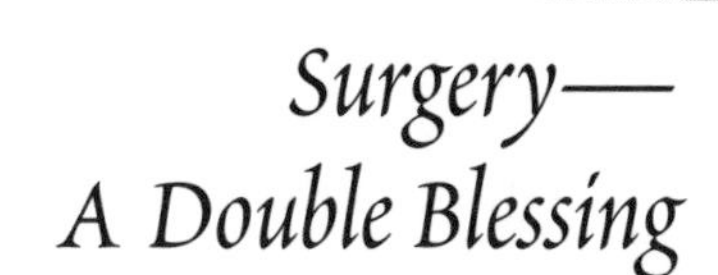

Chapter Six

Surgery—A Double Blessing

Before surgery on the day of my mastectomy, I asked the hospital chaplain to pray with me. After she left I felt a presence at the foot of my bed. It was nothing I could see, but it was so comforting and so peaceful. This was a major turning point for me. After that, I was never scared, angry, or upset. I had no fears whatever, not even of dying. After surgery, I had no pain and could even reach my arm all the way up above my head and squeeze the doctor's hand real hard. Before the mastectomy I was a believer in God and Jesus, but I am more emotional about religion now. I feel closer to God, with a real sense of comfort, as a result of the presence I felt that day.

Glenda

The Sunday before I was to have my double mastectomy, we attended church and our Sunday School class. By this time, the news was out—they knew that the lump was malignant. I can't describe the sense of caring and fellowship I experienced as so many people, men and women alike, embraced me.

Their promise to pray for me took the burden from me and divided it many times over. "You're in our prayers, Pam. We'll be praying for you tomorrow. I know God will take care of you. What time is your surgery? I'll pray for you at that specific time."

What a comfort this was to me and to Tom. We needed this prayer support and were grateful to everyone who was willing to ask for God's strength and peace and to tell us that they were there for us.

> *Other people's prayers have been like a prayer bath—lifting me out of the mire of despondency or self-pity that can happen with a diagnosis of breast cancer.*
>
> ***Kory***

Surgery was scheduled for 10:30 Monday morning, November 28. We were to arrive by 8:30 for check-in and routine work-ups. Our city had been inundated with a 12-inch snowfall on Sunday, so I was afraid traffic would be tied up all the way to the hospital. It wasn't, but I didn't want to take any chances. This was the day I had been waiting for since my biopsy. We left home at 6:45 and arrived an hour early, no delays, no backed-up traffic. Everything flowed smoothly.

While lying on the gurney in the surgical prep room, clad in the customary hospital gown and covered with thin hospital blankets, I was asked to sign the consent form. Fortunately, I noticed that it only mentioned a single mastectomy. "This is wrong. I'm supposed to have a double mastectomy. This only says right breast. Now what?" I asked the nurse.

"You'll have to wait for Dr. Hill. Good thing you noticed. I was just going to start your IV so you would've been a bit too groggy to say anything to him," the nurse anesthetist explained. "We'll wait till you've had a chance to talk to him. I'm sure he'll be here shortly."

Before I knew it, Dr. Hill was by my side. "Papers not right?" he asked.

I reminded him of his promise to do a double mastectomy.

"No problem, Pam, no problem at all."

The papers were quickly changed, I signed them, and I was on my way. I learned later that a friend had tried to get a double mastectomy only to be turned down by her insurance company. I was glad this decision was between Dr. Hill and me—where it belonged.

The three-hour surgery went well. It didn't hurt as much as I thought it would, or at least the medication did a good job of masking the pain.

Tom and I had to wait until Wednesday for the pathology report. I woke up that day thinking that things would be okay. I still had some fear and apprehension, but I had an underlying confidence that we would get a good report.

Dr. Hill entered my room with a big grin on his face. "I have your pathology report," he said. "I removed 22 lymph nodes and every one of them was clear—no sign of cancer. None!"

My husband and I were elated! "Thank you, Dr. Hill," we said at once. "Thank you!"

"But, wait till you hear this! We found in-situ cancer, actually a pre-cancerous condition in your left breast—the one you had me remove as a precaution." God's hand again.

"It was serendipitous that you had the other breast removed, Pam. Serendipitous!"

"Yes, it was," I agreed. But then I had to boldly proclaim, "I prefer to believe it was God acting in my life."

"That's one way of looking at it," he consented.

"Besides being the bearer of good news, I'm also here to take off your bandages," he said. "You don't need to look, and in fact, most women do not look at this point."

As he peeled away the white bandages that covered my entire chest, I lifted my head off the pillow to take a look. "I want to see," I assured him.

After all, I had seen my grandmother, pictures from Lyn, and my new friend Ann.

As I glanced down, I saw two long red lines across my chest. "Not bad, Dr. Hill. I can live with this. Dr. Hill," I continued, "I feel so fortunate, so very blessed!"

"You have a good attitude, Pam. That's not the usual reaction when the bandages are removed. I wish my other patients were as positive as you."

And indeed, I was ecstatic—nearly giddy! All the tension I had felt over not knowing if the cancer had spread was now gone. This was like a second chance at life. The cancer had been removed and I was healthy again. I may be without breasts, but the cancer had been discovered early, there was no node involvement, and I was now on the road to recovery. By the grace of God!

He told the nurse to pull out three of the four drainage tubes I had coming out of my sides where breast tissue had been, then handed me a prescription for oral antibiotics and Tylenol 3.

"You're ready to go home today, Pam. The only exercise I want you to do at this point is to lift your arms up to the top of your head. No climbing the walls with your fingers yet. I'll see you for a follow-up visit in the clinic in one week or in my St. Paul office on Monday, whichever you prefer."

With tears welling up in my eyes and a smile that could have melted all the snow outside my hospital room, I took his hand in mine, looked into his eyes, and gave him a heartfelt, "Thank you." Not a lot of words, but said with gratitude and praise as I realized that Dr. Hill had been a gift from God. His aggressive approach to lump removal and his willingness to perform the additional mastectomy at my request saved me from having the cancer spread throughout my body, had we waited and watched.

Lyn had heard our good news too and came in to congratulate us. "I'm so happy for you!" she told us.

While waiting for my prescription, I called lots of people—everyone I could think of, actually. I was so excited, you would have thought

I had been declared a winner in Publisher's Clearing House—and yet I was a winner! I had emerged from a pit of fear to the freedom of excellent health and a positive prognosis for the future.

My elation was rubbing off on my new hospital roommate who had just had a mastectomy that morning. "I hope to meet you again someday," she said. "I couldn't help but overhear your conversation with Dr. Hill. I appreciate your positive outlook. I only hope to be able to react the same."

When I got home I wrote something for our Sunday School Christmas newsletter. I couldn't wait to let everyone know what a personal God we have and how He had attended to each detail of my ordeal. The people who had prayed for me deserved to know that their prayers had indeed been answered.

Here's what I shared:

REJOICE

Do not be anxious about anything, but in everything by prayer and petition, with thanksgiving, present your requests to God. And the peace of God, which transcends all understanding, will guard your hearts and your minds in Christ Jesus. (Philippians 4:6-7).

As I reflect on the rollercoaster ride of the last three weeks that resulted in my double mastectomy this week, I can honestly say that it is by the grace of God that I have not fallen apart. As a result of all your prayers, I have maintained a positive attitude, while watching in humbleness, as God has answered every request for help.

I would love to share all the details with you in person, but for now, let me list for you some of the ways in which God has directed and touched my life:

- *He has intervened so that my lump was found at an early stage.*
- *As a means of preparation for the diagnosis of cancer, and before I had any idea that I would be facing a double mastectomy, God brought two total strangers into my life who also had breast cancer and who offered their support in my time of need.*
- *He has given me a surgeon who is willing to do aggressive surgery.*
- *He has provided me with reading materials and a knowledgeable RN to help me make an informed decision.*
- *When I finally made my decision to have the double mastectomy, I had a burning desire to know exactly what I would look like after surgery. God again introduced me to a woman at the home of our grieving friends. She volunteered to show me her scars (I didn't even need to ask) and provided me with complete peace and conviction in my decision.*
- *But most of all, God has given me all of you as prayer warriors, intervening on my behalf, praying for healing, peace and competent medical support.*

Praise the Lord! God has shown me that He really cares about the details of my life. I have always known that God loves me and cares for me, but the specific kind of support and guidance I have had over the last couple of weeks has been incredible.

I hope that by my openness in sharing a very personal experience, you will see the loving hand of God who has never left my side. I pray that you also will know the Lord and His peace, the peace which Philippians 4:7 says, "transcends all understanding."

Thank you for your continued prayer support as I schedule a visit with an oncologist to see if further treatment is advised.

Chapter Seven

The Pathology Report

God didn't come into my life until I was in the hospital. And then He came in a BIG way!! That's when my spiritual journey started—after my surgery. Even though I had been a Christian all my life, I was an intellectual Christian. I had more of it here in my head than I had in my heart.

I still feel blessed. I still feel God is with me. So what if I have another round of cancer. So what. I don't know why I'm still here. I think as long as I am here I'm getting bolder about my witnessing to people. I'm getting more knowledgeable about the Bible so when people ask me questions, I can talk somewhat intelligently about Scripture and things that have happened to me. I can share my particular journey.

Sherry

On December 5 I decided I couldn't live with that one remaining drainage tube in me anymore. Enough of this nonsense—such a bother. Since I wasn't supposed to drive yet, I called my neighbor Paula to see if she could take me to Dr. Hill's St. Paul office to have him pull it out.

As I lay on his examining table, he checked out his handiwork. "You look good, Pam, speaking from a surgeon's point of view, of course."

"To tell the truth, Doctor, I think I look pretty good, too. A little like an adolescent—not much different looking than a girl of 10 or 12."

"Actually, missing my breasts is not as bad as the reason for their removal. The cancer bothered me a whole lot more than the thought of being without breasts," I told him.

He pulled out the remaining tube. It felt good not to have that thing hanging from my side.

"Why don't you get dressed and then we can discuss your pathology report. It's ready for us to go over."

Sitting in his office, he looked at me with hesitation and apprehension as he began, "The best news, as I explained in the hospital, is that all 22 of your lymph nodes were negative. Other tests were done as well, and although yours were not bad, they were not exactly what we had hoped they would be."

"Your hormone receptors were negative—positive would've been better. Cells were abnormal—normal would've been better. Cells were growing at an intermediate rate—slow would've been better."

Of course, he explained this information in more detail, but at that point, I wasn't hearing the details.

All the joy I had felt over having negative lymph nodes now seemed to be swallowed up in news I was not prepared to accept. I felt like I'd just been hit a death blow. I wanted to leave his office, sit in a corner and cry. I was devastated.

My mouth went dry and my eyes filled with tears as I began to realize that I would now be a candidate for chemotherapy. I had been hoping that chemo wouldn't have been needed. I had never expected such bad news.

"I'm going to refer your records to Dr. Drake, an oncologist here in St. Paul. He's excellent. He will discuss these results in more detail and then decide a course of treatment for your particular needs," he explained.

I sincerely thanked Dr. Hill for all he had done for me and then immediately rushed to the breast center. I needed to talk to Lyn and show her these results. I had to get her perspective on what this all meant.

I handed Lyn the report. She explained terminology that was not at all familiar and assured me that Dr. Drake was indeed an excellent oncologist. He had recently completed a fellowship in oncology at a well-known cancer center, which meant he would be up-to-date on all the latest treatments. That was reassuring information that I needed to hear.

Despite Lyn's words of encouragement, I couldn't hold back the tears any longer. I sat on the waiting room couch, with Paula by my side, and wept uncontrollably. The anxiety over my future was combined for the first time with a sense of self-pity. I felt as if my entire world was about to collapse.

I was glad they didn't tell me to "lighten up" or look at the positive side as people tend to do in situations like mine. They let me do what I needed to do—sit there with a handful of tissues and just cry.

I'm sure I looked a fright, but I didn't care. I was releasing a mountain of sadness that I had held onto since my initial diagnosis.

> *My husband was just wonderful. He never told me I shouldn't feel the way I felt. If I told him I just felt like crying or I just felt like being grouchy, he'd tell me that was fine, I could do that. He never made it difficult for me to work my way through what was going on. He was and is supportive to the "nth" degree.*
>
> ***Julia***

The tears seemed to cleanse some of the grief and pain from my spirit. I felt better as Paula and I stood to leave. I thanked Lyn for explaining my report to me and for letting me be myself with her.

Paula drove me home and we sat in her car for a while in my driveway. "Thank you for being with me today Paula, for letting me be myself and for listening to my fears." I wept again. I seemed to be absorbed in self-pity. I guess it was about time to own up to the fact that I had undergone major surgery for breast cancer. Despite all the good that had happened, it was a life-threatening situation and there was plenty to make me feel nervous and upset, for a short while anyway. I did not want to get stuck feeling sorry for myself, but I needed to acknowledge that this was not an easy path.

Once in the privacy of my own home, I let down my guard completely and cried again. When Tom returned from work, he took one look at me and knew something was wrong. In his understanding and compassionate way, he drew me to him and wrapped his big strong arms around my shaking body. I still believed that I was very blessed that the cancer was found early. Very fortunate!

But for now, for today, I cried!!!!

> *I just know that God is taking care of me. And it's not that I don't have great rounds of fear, because I do. I'm very human. I do still have days, not so much anymore, but in January I had to have a CAT scan. So there was anxiety and fear. Would they find something?*
>
> ***Sherry***

That evening after dinner, I again realized that God had actually prepared me for chemotherapy. On the preceding Saturday I had had a visit from a woman I had come to know the previous year when I taught in a program that served students who had dropped out of high school. Mary and I didn't know each other well, but I had learned that she had had a mastectomy and was a breast cancer survivor. She was open about her experience and seemed very positive, talking about her progress to staff who knew her well. Mary seemed to have adjusted well to her circumstances and even joked about how we couldn't even guess which one of her breasts was real.

As we sat sipping tea in my dark kitchen on a cloudy autumn Saturday morning, Mary asked, "Would you like to see my prosthesis?" Her nonchalance was welcome. No modesty, no embarrassment. Just a willingness to help me along on my journey, even more than either of us was aware of at that moment. As she reached under her blouse, she removed a soft, warm, silicone breast as if she were removing a ribbon from her hair. "Here, you can hold it if you like." And I did, no problem. I know some women are totally devastated by the loss of a breast, but that was not my reaction. I was born with a less-than-perfect body. Life mattered more to me than appearance.

"Did you know I needed to have chemotherapy?" she asked. "Would you also like to see where they placed my catheter?" She showed me a small bump above her remaining breast. A central catheter is like a stainless steel two-inch cube with a rubber center and a plastic tube extending from it. The cube is placed about four inches below the collarbone, under the skin, and then the tubing is threaded into the heart artery. All the chemotherapy nurse needs to do is locate the center rubber section that is about the size of a dime, stick an IV needle in it with a plastic tube attached, and the patient is ready to begin a chemotherapy treatment.

Mary explained that she had undergone her treatments at home in the comfort of her lounge chair. "If you like, I can give you the name of the people I used. I'm sure they could accommodate you too," she offered. "Your insurance company would most likely provide this service. That is, if you need chemo."

"Nice of you to give me all this information," I thought. Along with my polite words was a cocky confidence that I would not need chemo. I did not need to know the details of a catheter, but I could listen and be polite. I told myself that I would tuck this knowledge away and share it someday with someone less fortunate than myself. I was healed. I had survived surgery. There was no lymph node involvement, no need for me to do anything additional. Or so I thought.

Actually, when I thought further about her selection of home treatment, I realized that if I were in Mary's situation, I would prefer to have my treatments in a public place. "I like the company of others," I told her. "It helps me feel less scared if I know in the cubicle or room right next to me there are people just like me getting treatment." I had a feeling of camaraderie for people I did not know, but who, like me, were getting chemo. I wanted to be around these people. "I'm glad that method worked for you," I told her. "Thanks for the suggestion."

Mary did confess that despite the comfort of being treated in her own home, there was also a disadvantage. She explained that once her chemo was completed, she didn't even want to look at the chair she had sat in for those treatments. It was a source of comfort then; now it was a reminder, right in her own home, of the cancer she had hoped was behind her.

When our visit was over, I thanked Mary for her openness and her willingness to share with me. I did not know it at the time of her visit, but God was again attending to the details, preparing me for chemotherapy and the catheter I would need.

It wasn't until I was alone in my bedroom, filled with anxiety over my need for further treatment, that I began to reflect on this time alone with Mary. She was a real live person with the same experience as mine. I wasn't alone. What comfort this was for me to know someone who had walked the path I was about to walk. And she had survived!

It was as if God were telling me, "Look at her. Listen to her. She survived. So will you."

After I realized what God had done for me, this practical, caring God, I felt confident that with God's help I could beat this disease.

> *I felt that the Lord was bringing people into my life that He wanted me to share with. There was a young woman getting chemo the same time I was. She asked my husband which one of us was getting chemo, because neither of us looked ill. I told her I was. She told me I looked too happy. She would call me and tell me her fears. It just seemed that there was this contact between us. I brought her into my prayer life and started praying for her. We called each other and I shared my faith and encouragement with her.*
>
> **Elaine**

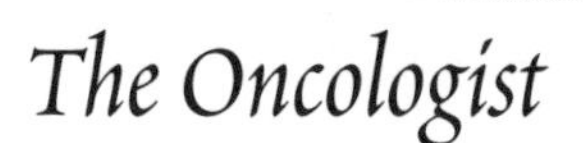

Chapter Eight

The Oncologist

I went to my oncologist's office to talk about the upcoming events. I was very fearful and I said, "God, I'm just going to sit in here and I'm going to pray. I'll pray for myself." I was very self-oriented.

When I got into that waiting room, it was full! It was packed! I'd love to walk into an oncologist's office and have no one there. They would go out of business because no one would have cancer. That's my biggest prayer!

I sat down on the chair, looked around and thought, "These are all God's people. Each and every one of them. And they're hurting."

And I thought, "Who's praying for them?"

I sat there and I prayed for every person in that office. I was filled with God's love and His compassion. It wasn't like me. It really touches me because that was powerful for me that day. Because I was so self-oriented and God just took ***the me*** *out of it and said, "Look around."*

It was a wonderful experience when I sat there and prayed for all those people. For whatever reason, I'm sure God put that on my heart.

Sherry

On December 6 Tom and I went to see my oncologist, Dr. Drake. I was immediately impressed by the kindness of his staff. They all seemed to smile and be extremely patient. No one looked rushed or irritated with anyone. I imagined that they had received special training in how to interact with cancer patients.

As I sat down to complete new patient forms, I looked around the waiting room—not too many people. I noticed another woman about my age filling out forms. What was her story? Did she also have breast cancer? I was always curious about what was happening to other people. Unlike my initial experience in Dr. Hill's office where I felt like I didn't belong, I knew I belonged here, and I felt sympathy and compassion for these people who were just like me. We shared a common disease—cancer, and a common goal—the hope for healing.

In walked a tall, muscular, nice-looking young man, about 23, I guess. He was bald and had a red bandanna around his head and a baseball cap over that. Telltale sign of why we were all there.

I observed an elderly couple. I guessed that she was the one with cancer. Was it the wig that gave her away?

All in all, it was not a sad place, just a new place for us.

"Pam," the nurse called, "you may see Dr. Drake now."

"Can my husband come, too?" I asked.

"After you've talked to Dr. Drake alone. He likes to talk to his patients before the family joins in," she explained.

Dr. Drake's desk was stacked high with patient charts. He had my chart opened. "Hello, Pam. I'm Dr. Drake. Please have a seat. I'd like to start to get to know you. Why don't you begin by telling me a bit about yourself."

Having breast cancer was making me very bold in my witness, so I began by telling him I was a Christian. "I can see God's hand in all that's happened to me. All the details, from pre-diagnosis, to the removal of the left breast which unexpectedly had cancer, to God putting total strangers in my life to comfort and encourage me. All these details have been worked out by God," I told him.

He listened patiently, as if he had all day. "I find everyone's story interesting. As you can see by my desk, I hear a lot of stories."

"Now, let's get technical for a while and go over your pathology report. I've called the lab to have the biopsy results sent to me. I have the mastectomy report right here, but I also want to see what the biopsy showed."

"First of all, your hormone receptor is negative. If it had been positive, you could have taken Tamoxifen. This is a drug that is believed to play a role in cancer prevention. But don't worry about that. The size of your tumor was 1.5 cm—about 3/4 inch. At 1 cm. we do not believe chemo is necessary. At 2 we definitely recommend it. The tumor was not slow growing and not fast—it is intermediate. The cancer cells were not normal looking (sounded like an oxymoron to me) and not wildly distorted. They were sort of distorted."

"I never suspected that there would be this much to know about a tumor. I thought a tumor was a tumor. You removed it, and that was that. I was never aware of all this analysis," I told him.

"You are in the mid range on all these indicators, Pam. Because of that, I recommend that you have chemotherapy. Your prognosis is excellent. In fact, 85 percent of breast cancer patients with a report like yours have no recurrence. If you decide to have the chemo, that will add 4-5 percent. We hit the body hard with the drugs for about four months."

He went on to talk about three chemotherapy drugs. Two of them were standard procedure and used for most cases of breast cancer. For the third drug there was a choice between two kinds. One is pretty hard on the heart and can weaken it later in life. This drug causes you to lose your hair. He said there is another drug that is about as effective, maybe 1 percent less so, but not as hard on the system. He said the percentage difference between the two drugs is almost negligible. "I'd recommend the drug with fewer side effects for you," he explained. "For your particular case, I believe it's the best choice."

We also discussed my poor veins and how my IV had leaked into my arm following surgery. He said that was another reason for going with the second drug, because if the other one were to leak out of my vein it would cause major problems. The side effects did not warrant a mere 1 percent increase in effectiveness. Besides, how does one measure this anyway?

I felt good about his decision—our decision.

He had me go across the hall where the chemotherapy is given. "Go talk to Joan. She's an oncology nurse who can look at your veins and see if she agrees that a central catheter is the way to go. She'll show you one and explain how it works."

Joan was a very pleasant nurse who greeted me with a warm smile. Like the staff in Dr. Drake's office, the staff in the chemo area seemed to have such pleasant personalities—loaded with patience, understanding and a kind of laid-back attitude.

Joan examined the veins in my left arm and agreed that these tiny veins were no match for the chemotherapy. (I had had the lymph nodes removed from under my right arm, which meant that I was never to have any more injections, including chemotherapy, in that arm.) Although there was no need to remove the lymph nodes from my left side, the veins in that arm were smaller than normal due to being born without a left hand. Two arms, but neither one suitable for the chemo.

"I think you are an excellent candidate for the catheter. Tell Dr. Drake that I agree with his recommendation," said Joan.

Back in Dr. Drake's office I noticed his Fellowship in Oncology certificate that Lyn had mentioned. It means he's up-to-date on cancer. GOOD! After my physical exam it was time to bring Tom in on the conversation.

Dr. Drake filled Tom in on the plan to do chemotherapy. He told Tom that a good indicator of how I would do related to my experience with morning sickness when I was pregnant. "If you got sick then, you are apt to have a rougher time. If not, it should not be a major problem."

"I'm relieved. I had almost no morning sickness with either pregnancy," I told him.

As for my hair, the drug that he recommended, the one less harsh on my system, would not cause my hair to fall out completely. "You might have some hair loss, but not total," he said.

Tom and I had previously discussed buying a wig. I had told him that if I were going to lose my hair, I would buy the most beautiful red wig I could find. I had always admired redheads, and now I could be one. But with Dr. Drake's prediction, I figured I wasn't going to need a wig after all. Good news.

Before I left his office I had two appointments. The first was 7:30 Monday morning for Dr. Hill to insert the catheter, and the second for the first chemotherapy treatment to follow at 10:30.

I left Dr. Drake's office that day convinced of three things: 1) He was an expert on treating cancer; 2) I would have minimal problems with chemotherapy; and 3) I could look forward to an excellent prognosis. I had been given a very important ingredient on my way to recovery: HOPE.

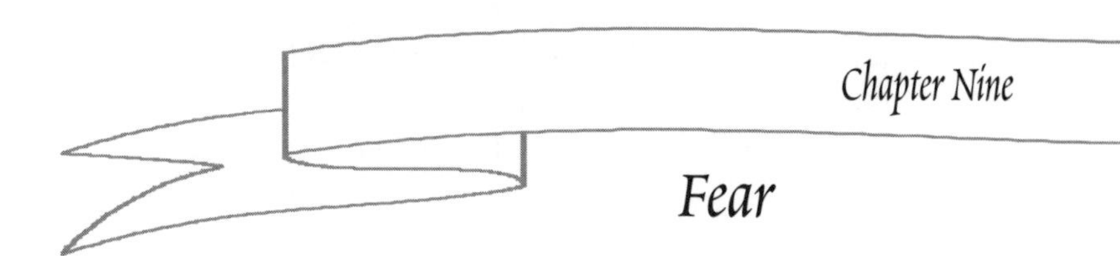

Chapter Nine

Fear

When I reflect on it, there were times when I had some despair. At one point I even called my pastor and asked him for advice on how to cope with despondency. That's kind of how I felt.

Kory

At one time I felt so low, so down, like the fiddler in 'Fiddler on the Roof.' I asked, "Hey, Lord, remember me?" It isn't wrong to feel that way, to have fear. But He will overcome it for you, if you can pray to the Lord.

Elaine

I needed to see Dr. Hill for follow-up and have him remove some tiny strips of tape from my chest as well as discuss how I was progressing since surgery. It was also a good time for us to talk about my need for chemo and how he would insert the central catheter.

"All I do is numb you up a bit and then place the catheter right below your collarbone. I'll thread a tube to your heart and you'll be all set to go. That way the chemotherapy drugs can go where they're supposed to, and it won't be so hard on your veins. I'll do this at 7:30 a.m. in the hospital. Then you can go right next door to the clinic for your first treatment at 10:30."

"By the way, I know I had originally thought you might not need chemo. But I agree with Dr. Drake's advice. He's the oncologist, the expert on breast cancer. How old are you?" he asked.

"I'm 46."

"Well," he said, "we're the same age. I certainly know I would do the same thing if I were in your shoes. My advice—go for it!"

"I intend to. But I have a question. I feel pretty good, but I'm still in a lot of pain. Is that normal? I guess the drugs I got in the hospital did a good job of masking the pain."

"Yes, perfectly normal. It's a painful operation, Pam. You've only been out of surgery for nine days."

He renewed my Tylenol 3 prescription because it's good to have on hand for my pain. I asked for a prosthesis prescription, even though I wasn't sure of my decision to buy them yet. He said I'd probably want them and maybe would want reconstruction. I wasn't sure I wanted anything at this point. I had even jokingly told my 10-year-old daughter that because I didn't have breasts now, I could go topless at the beach.

You should have seen the look on her face!

Two church friends dropped off dinner that evening. Throughout my recovery and treatment time we were blessed with numerous delicious meals, many of which, as it turned out, were chicken breasts. We laughed over the irony of people bringing us breasts, when I had lost mine. This may seem a bit bizarre, but we looked for humor anywhere we could find it.

A friend from work came to see me after dinner. My husband and daughter had gone to church, so we were able to have a nice long chat. She brought spring flowers, two purple irises, and said she was tired of winter, even if it hadn't officially started. I loved those flowers because they were a reminder of the beauty God has given us as well as the promise of spring.

The next morning at 8:45 a neighbor delivered that evening's dinner. "Put it in the oven at 275 degrees for five hours," he instructed. It was a delicious beef stew with carrots, potatoes, peas, lots of onion, celery and gravy. Included were two bags of cookies, grain muffins, and a delicious loaf of pumpkin bread. Again and again we were blessed with the many meals that were brought to our door.

My folks came over for a while in the afternoon. They drove me around to do some errands. I didn't have a lot of energy yet, but I had enough to finish my Christmas shopping. This was probably the earliest I'd ever been completely ready for the holidays.

They also drove me to my office to say hello. It was so good to see everybody and to fill them in on my progress. I was showered with words of encouragement and warm, firm embraces as people put their arms around me in love. What comfort I found in their touch.

I told them I was hoping to be back to work by Tuesday. That was my goal. I'm not the kind of person who relaxes easily. I like to have something to do, and once I began to feel better, I figured I was better off at work, being busy, than moping around the house worrying about myself.

Our son Peter was home from college for Christmas break, so all four of us enjoyed the beef stew that had been cooking in the oven all day. It tasted as good as it smelled.

After dinner we went to hear our daughter's friend perform at her first Christmas concert. It felt good to get out and be around people again in a setting other than my home or the hospital. We even went to the Dairy Queen after the concert. It was so fun. Half the kids from the concert were there, giggling and acting like typical ten year olds. It had been a long time since we'd had a good laugh. It felt refreshing.

Despite the attempt at getting my life back to normal, going to concerts, eagerly looking forward to returning to work, and finishing my Christmas shopping, I was constantly aware that I was facing chemo.

I talked to Joan, the oncology nurse, about my fear of having a bad reaction. I told her how my dad and I had discussed our preference to just get the treatment that we knew we needed, not asking about possible side effects. We feared getting a reaction just because it was possible or, if not getting it, being too apprehensive to continue the treatment that we knew we needed.

"There's a video you can watch before your first treatment. I think this will help you tremendously. It shows several different people being treated with chemotherapy, yet maintaining active lifestyles. I think you'll be encouraged. Also, I'll respect your wishes and not tell you anything you don't need to know. Some patients want to know all the details. Others are like you."

"I don't mind knowing that I'll experience fatigue and nausea. Anything else scares me," I explained.

That evening I confided in Tom. "I'm so nervous. I'm really afraid of chemo. I'm anxious about side effects. I know Dr. Drake doesn't expect anything horrible to happen, but what if something does?"

"Whoa! Calm down, Pam. Don't get yourself all worked up. I know you're scared, but I also know everything will turn out fine," he said as he tried to reassure me. "Why the sudden fear? I thought you were handling this pretty well after our talk with Dr. Drake."

"I was, but you know how it is when someone tells you not to look at something. What do you do? You look. Well, I had a book that told about chemotherapy. I was reading some sections when I came across the chapter on side effects. Well, I read a few and my mind started to think of all kinds of horrible possibilities happening to me."

"Come here, Pam." Tom reached for me, placing my limp, shaking body next to his. There wasn't anything he could say to set my mind at ease. But the warmth of his arms around me and the comfort I felt with my head snuggled into his chest made me feel loved and cared for, which I needed more than anything else at this time.

"I'm scared, Tom, just plain scared. I need God's help more than ever. What I really fear is fear. What if I am so overcome with fear that I decide not to get the treatments. Then what?"

But wait a minute! I remembered my conversation with another mom at the concert that evening. She had told me that same day was the funeral of a fifth grader's father. He had died of a brain tumor. I think this was God's way of telling me to do all I could do. I still had a chance that father didn't.

I knew what I needed to do. I needed to do the chemo, but I needed the peace of God so I wouldn't panic.

In the safety of Tom's continued embrace I cried. I did feel bad about what was happening to me. When I was able to be light-hearted it was easier. I wanted to be cheerful, but I couldn't. Not at that moment.

The next day, December 10, I got up early to make breakfast. The phone rang and it was our pastor.

"How are you doing, Pam?"

"Let me be honest, Pastor. I'm not doing so well. I'm scared of chemo. I know I need it, but I'm afraid."

He could sense the despair in my voice. Tears began to fall as he said, "You know, Pam. I was wondering when you were going to crash. You have had such a positive attitude all along. I was wondering when reality was going to set in."

"Well, it's happened. I've crashed. I'm not so positive anymore."

"Can I pray for you over the phone, Pam?" my pastor asked?

"Please...I need that," I said haltingly.

"God, protect Pam with your angels. Surround her with your love and compassion. She's hurting now, God. Be her constant companion in this difficult period of her life. Amen."

"Yes, God, surround me with your angels," I thought.

God's timing was perfect. My sad spirit began to fade as I was prayed for over the phone. How simple and yet what an effect it had on me.

> *For about a year after my diagnosis, I didn't know how to pray. So a friend of mine called the Carmelite nuns in Hudson, Wisconsin. They prayed for me round the clock. If I woke up at 2 a.m. it was comforting to know that a nun was praying for me at that very moment. I believe prayer was one of the nicest gifts I got.*
>
> **Nini**

That day as I knelt to pray by the side of my bed, I put my hands palms up and heard birds singing. I was reminded of how God cares for the birds.

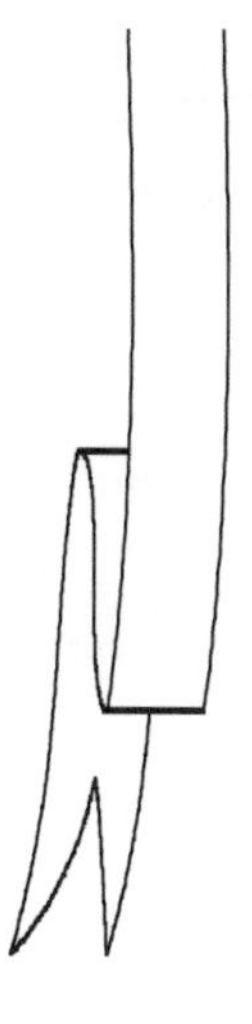

"Consider the ravens:

They do not sow or reap,
they have no storeroom or barn;

yet God feeds them.

And how much more valuable
you are than birds!"

LUKE 12:24

A friend and I went for a walk at Woodlake Nature Center. We saw three baby fox wrestling, playing and pushing each other off the walkway. They were probably 25 feet away from us. The smallest of them, about 6-8 inches tall, came trotting over to us. When it got about five feet away, he cocked his head one way, and then the other and looked at me. It was really as if God were telling me through the fox, "I'm one of His creatures, too. And He takes care of me and I know He'll take care of you." That was a wonderful experience.

Kory

Surely He will care for me. He will see me through this trial, not with my strength but with His. I'm not as strong as I lead others to believe. It was time for me to completely rely on God's strength.

That afternoon my good friend Kory came to visit. Our purpose was to write out our Christmas cards together. I had my supplies ready to go when she walked in with a large cloth bag full of her Christmas cards and address books. I played a tape of Christian songs and put on a pot of water for hot tea. As we conveyed our Christmas greetings, I realized what a precious gift Kory was to me. Here she was, in the middle of the busy Christmas season, spending unhurried time with me. No hustle bustle or words of, "Oh, I should get going. I have so much to do." She was there for me. It was one of my favorite afternoons of my recovery.

At one point, as I was relishing the good time we were having, I took her hand in mine and confessed, "You know, Kory, I'm not strong. This is very hard for me to deal with. I'm just not strong."

I think I needed to confess to someone that my lightheartedness was disappearing. I needed to be honest about my feelings.

Kory responded perfectly in her understanding and compassionate way when she said, "Who is? Who is strong?"

Exactly! We don't need to be strong. Our strength is in the Lord. It was such a comfort to hear her say that. I didn't need to be a "super" woman. I could admit to others that I was having a hard time. In my weakness, God's strength is seen.

On Sunday, December 11, my pastor came up to me, took my hand and said, "I'm still praying for your fear to be gone."

"I think it's working, Pastor. I'm beginning to feel better. I'm amazingly calm."

I, too, was praying for God's protection from fear. I knew I had cancer and that I needed treatment, but I was so scared of being scared.

It was at this point that I recalled my conversation with a woman from church. She told me she had several friends who had recently had mastectomies and then chemo. One woman in particular had breezed through her treatment.

Breezed through! Again, I saw this as a message from God telling me I would be all right. If other women could come out okay, so could I. Concrete proof like this was exactly what I needed to calm me down.

Now I could face tomorrow. I could face chemo.

When I was in the hospital a friend came and gave me a Precious Moments figure. It said, "Time heals." And it was almost like God sent that person that day to give me that gift so I would finally get my act together and go forward. It was the timing of her visit and the timing of the gift. It was perfect.

Nini

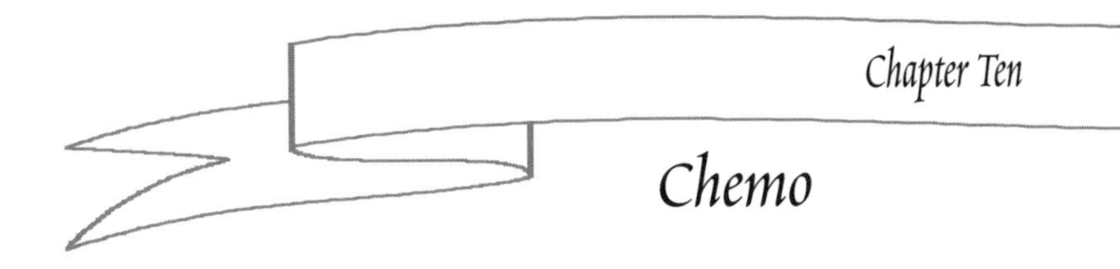

Chapter Ten

Chemo

On Monday morning, December 12, we arrived at the hospital at 5:40—ten minutes later than my scheduled time. This was significant for me, since it was concrete proof that I was not in a nervous tizzy. Usually I'm at least half an hour early for hospital appointments.

After I checked in at the front desk, I was told to report to the sixth floor. I changed into the standard hospital attire: drafty blue print gown, stretchy slippers and terrycloth robe. I sat down in the chair and started to crochet while I waited for the nurse to call my name.

"You look like you live here, Pam," Tom said.

"I'm truly relaxed, at peace about the chemo now," I assured him.

Dr. Hill arrived late. He thought the surgery was scheduled for 8:00 and not 7:30.

"Don't worry about it, Doctor. I checked with Joan last week and she assured me that whatever time I finish in surgery, I can still get my treatment. That's all I care about. I'm ready to begin today."

"While you're at it, would you mind smoothing out my incisions a bit? I seem to have a slight pucker on my left side and a 'blob' under my right arm."

"Oh, that's what we call a 'dog ear'. I'd be glad to fix those two spots for you," he said.

That's what I liked about Dr. Hill. He was kind, respectful and accommodating. If I was going to be flat, I wanted my flatness to look good. He did that for me and I was grateful.

The catheter was inserted with no problem. Although the device was a God-send and would make my chemo treatments uneventful, it took me several weeks to get used to this stainless steel box being in my chest. It was very difficult to get comfortable in bed. I eventually learned to prop pillows in such a way that it eased the discomfort I felt.

Once the catheter was in place I got dressed and was then wheeled to the chemo office. There were ten chairs in the waiting room, all lined up against a glass wall. Immediately behind the waiting room was a large room divided off by cubicles, much like a business office. Each cubicle had two chairs, one for the patient and one for a guest, as well as all the standard equipment the nursing staff would need to administer the treatment. Beyond the cubicles and along the outside wall were about five private treatment rooms complete with a recliner, a television, a telephone and a window. These rooms were used for people whose treatments took the longest.

Tom and I started out in a cubicle. It was a busy day with a lot of people getting treated. The nurse began to explain what she was going to do. We were then taken to the conference room where we watched an excellent video on people receiving chemo—the one Joan had previously mentioned. Each person in this film took their treatments in stride. They kept up their regular activities, remained at work and generally led normal lives. This video made me feel like I could handle the chemo and that my life with its routines and pleasures would remain basically the same.

After the video was completed, one of the outside rooms became available. I was ready to begin the first of six treatments.

"I'm going to start you out by giving you something to drink, Pam. We have pop, coffee, Postum or hot chocolate. Anything sound good to you? It's important to drink a lot of liquid when you're being treated. Including at home, too," she instructed.

"I'll try Postum," I said. "That's something new for me. I'll be adventurous."

"Okay. Now let's get down to business. Let me see where Dr. Hill put your central catheter," she said, as I opened my blouse to show her.

"Oh, that's excellent! It protrudes from your chest just right. We'll have no trouble giving you your chemo through this. You know, some doctors bury the catheter so it is hardly accessible. Dr. Hill did a great job for you!"

"I'm glad to hear that."

She wiped off the skin covering the catheter with iodine and then stuck in the needle and tubing that would be used for the treatment. It didn't even hurt.

"I'm going to begin by giving you a bag of anti-nausea medication in an IV drip. This will take about half an hour. Then I'll come back and give you two of the chemo drugs in shot form. The third one I'll give you as an IV."

"We'll let this third drug drip in slowly. Otherwise, your face could get hot if it goes in too fast."

"Good idea," I said. "Thanks for telling me."

Having a hot face made me nervous. I don't know why. All I know is I tried to avoid anything abnormal. I'd stay there all day if it meant my face wouldn't feel weird. On a scale of 1 to 10, a hot face is nothing, but it was one thing I could control in this uncontrollable position.

With treatment number one completed, Tom and I went home. I felt fine. I had a tuna sandwich for lunch and just took it easy the rest of the afternoon. I got a call from our church organist who had had breast cancer five years before. It was nice talking to someone who knew how I felt. She told me that she usually stayed around home the day of treatment, but then returned to work the next day. That was encouraging news for me to know that I'd be able to work the next day.

A friend from church delivered dinner that evening.

"What do you suppose she brought us?" I asked Tom as we unveiled the foil covering.

"Huge chicken breasts, the largest ones I've ever seen!" exclaimed Tom. We looked at each other and burst out laughing!

I ate slowly. I was starting to get a queasy stomach. I had a metallic taste in my mouth—a reaction that I had been told might happen. I ate what I could of this delicious dinner, but the taste of metal came through.

"I'm sorry, but I just can't eat any more. I need to lie down," I said, as I excused myself to the family room couch.

I soon excused myself again and decided to go to bed. I took an anti-nausea pill, a pain pill and tried to get to sleep. I had a terrible headache!

I awoke the next morning at five, took my medications, and was ready to begin the day. In fact I felt so good that I got up and decided to take my dog out for a stroll. This was the beginning of a new life. I was determined to demonstrate a positive attitude. Walking in the pre-dawn hours was something I had never done before and it felt great! This was the new me!

In addition to regular exercise, I decided to pay particular attention to my eating habits, another area where I could have some control. I had read that a diet low in fat, full of fresh fruits and vegetables, particularly the ones containing anti-oxidant vitamins could perhaps prevent cancer.

I had intended for this to be my first day back at work. I had felt good during my walk, but once I got home and took my shower I felt lightheaded. I decided to stay home and allow my body to have the rest it was telling me it needed. I called work and said I would be starting back the next day instead. They understood completely.

I spent the entire day snuggled in bed, dozing off and on and reading magazines. I hadn't realized how exhausted I was, both physically and mentally. Fortunately our son Peter was still home from college so he took good care of me, bringing me breakfast and lunch in bed. Dry Apple Cinnamon Cheerios and orange juice seemed to settle my stomach and a hearty portion of good old macaroni and cheese made for a pleasant lunch, despite the metal taste in my mouth.

I was able to return to work the next day—accompanied by soda crackers and grape pop. All I had missed was two weeks and two days. Not bad for a double mastectomy!

Before I left for work, Joan, the chemo nurse, called to see how I was doing. She reassured me that I would do just fine on chemo. "You may get a bit more tired for a longer period of time, but that's all you can probably expect. You will not get sicker with additional treatments, so don't worry about that." I thanked her for her encouragement.

I repeated those words to myself. "You will not get sicker. You will not get sicker."

For the rest of the treatments I brought along a friend or I went alone. I specifically told my husband that it wasn't necessary for him to be with me. I know he would have been by my side, had I asked, but I decided to do this without him. My choice. I wanted our life to go back to a regular routine and having him at work made my life seem normal. I also didn't want any unnecessary fuss.

I found that talkative friends were good company. They helped pass the time (about three hours) and keep my mind off the chemo. When friends weren't available, I brought along a good book and lots of magazines. I was usually fortunate to get one of those small private rooms with a TV, another helpful distraction. My goal was to focus on positive thoughts and think of the chemo as a short path I had to take on my road to recovery.

Joan's prediction held true. Each treatment was pretty much the same: a metallic taste, a headache around supper time, and a slightly queasy stomach. This was as bad as it ever got for me. I never once vomited! Never! Amazing!

In fact, immediately after I completed my treatments, all of which were in the morning, (except the first one) I went to my part-time job. Armed with soda crackers and grape pop or Sprite, I found that I could work for four hours. This was very important to me. I needed to prove to myself that my whole life did not revolve around this disease and its treatments.

I decided that my final treatment deserved some fanfare. I bought two glass candy bowls, one for Dr. Drake's office and one for the chemo station and filled them with peppermints, a favorite of chemo patients. I offered these presents with a heartfelt "thanks" for the care I had received. These people helped me through the most difficult experience of my life and I wanted them to know how much their words of encouragement and hope had meant to me. I had made it through six treatments, even though at the beginning I had feared I would not even be able to start. By the grace of God!

Praise the Lord! I survived chemo!

> *Lois and I have a support group for cancer survivors. We give out a prayer jar that is called "prescriptions" of prayer. Members are to take one a day for encouragement. We even send these to other people we pray for around the country. We also give out a poem by Helen Steiner Rice entitled "The End of the Road Is But a Bend in the Road." It's such a beautiful poem because sometimes you do feel that it's the end of the road. It's just a bend.*
>
> **Nini**

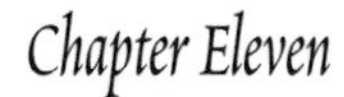

A Watched Over Life

My life will never be the same. It has changed for the better. I certainly would not have asked for the experience of breast cancer, but I know that having survived it, I can honestly say it has been good for my soul.

> *I bought a really bright-colored dress and also a short outfit at a garage sale. I don't recall that I've ever bought clothes for myself at a garage sale. Before I never even looked at them. My boss noticed that after the diagnosis I was cheerier, wore brighter colors and just seemed to grasp life more. I give a lot more hugs than I ever did because I know how much people mean to me. And I appreciate so much what people have done for me. So I think my relationships with people are different. I probably look at things on a little deeper level than I used to. I know how fragile life is. My husband and I have gotten closer. We were pretty close to begin with. And I've realized all the more how much I have to depend on Christ.*
>
> **Kory**

> *It really has changed my life. My friend Nini and I have said that even though we don't like living with cancer we feel we have changed so much we wouldn't want to go back to the per-*

son we were before. It's a change for the better. I'm much more aware, much more in tune. I have more empathy now than I did before. I appreciate life more. I'm now writing a book I had always wanted to write. I never would have written it, had I not been put in the position of now or never. So I think it opens up avenues for you that you might not have done otherwise. I have really started appreciating life. I can't tell you the number of times during the day that I thank God for something.

Lois

When I visit a breast cancer patient I tell them they are going to see many blessings out of this. They look at me as if I am a fool. But one of my blessings has been my new house. We bought this house because of my cancer. I thought, if my life is shortened, where do I want to live? The answer was, in the country. So my husband and I bought this house in the country. And a day doesn't go by that I don't thank God for life.

Nini

One of the things that we have always said is that our friendship has been so important to us. We never would have had this friendship (because our children are different ages and we belong to different churches) had it not been for our common experience of breast cancer. There is such a bond there. We've said it's like a sisterhood; there is such empathy with fellow breast cancer survivors.

We're much more outgoing and courageous. Nini heads a support group, took her son on a three-hour car trip, and even goes on water park rides, none of which she would have done before her diagnosis. Lois took a ride in a mountain gondola, despite her fear of heights. She was so proud of her accomplishment!

Lois and Nini

I have been blessed and God has been with me every minute of this whole situation. And it has grown my faith and brought me into a closer walk, a love relationship with God and Jesus Christ. I've come to know the Holy Spirit, which I knew nothing about before this cancer situation and studying the Bible.

Sherry

I guess what I need to say is, "Praise the Lord!" that He does things for us. I don't think I fully understand what having breast cancer has meant in my life, nor have I resolved all the issues that have come out of it. But I do feel that God has been with us and has held onto us whether we could or would or whatever. And it has been great that way. It's strengthened my faith a lot. It has strengthened my sense of security in the Lord's love for me.

Julia

I have come to understand that God really does love me and that He cares enough about me to send me help, sometimes before I even know I need it. As the Good Shepherd, He certainly tended to my every need. My first simple prayer, "God, may there be an understanding person at the clinic," was only the beginning of God's intervention of care and compassion for me as He took me by the hand and guided me every step of the way.

Clearly, the Lord watched over me. My prayer is that you will let Him do the same for you.

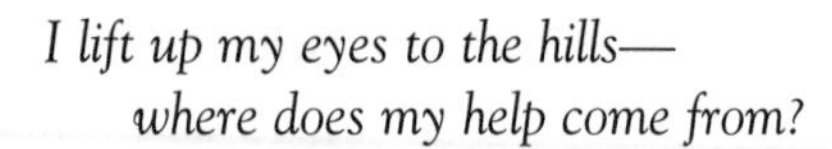

I lift up my eyes to the hills—
where does my help come from?

My help comes from the Lord,
the Maker of heaven and earth.

He will not let your foot slip—
he who watches over you will not slumber;
indeed; he who watches over Israel
will neither slumber nor sleep.

The Lord watches over you—
the Lord is your shade at your right hand;
the sun will not harm you by day,
nor the moon by night.

The Lord will keep you from all harm—
he will watch over your life;
the Lord will watch over your coming and
going both now and forevermore.

PSALM 121

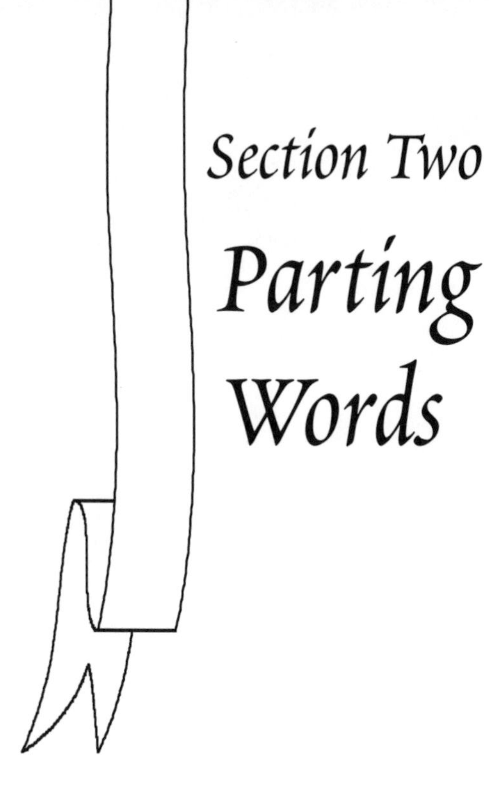

Section Two

Parting Words

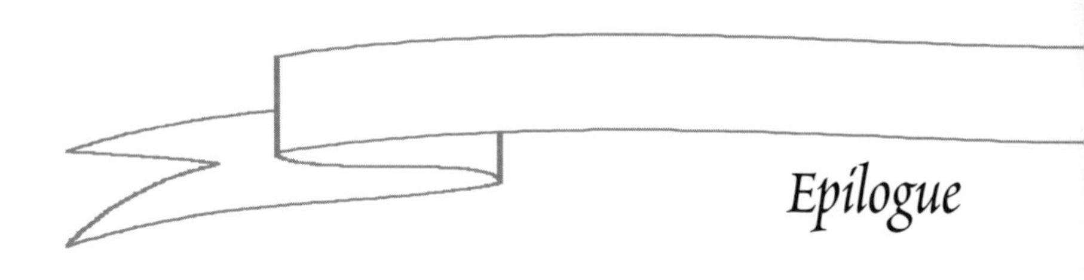

Epilogue

According to the American Cancer Society Breast Cancer Resource Center, excluding skin cancer, breast cancer is the most common form of cancer in women. The good news is that nearly 97% of women diagnosed at an early stage survive more than five years. This is why early detection is so important. I would encourage everyone to contact the American Cancer Society for more information on treatment options, prevention and care.

Since I had never had a life-threatening illness before, I handled it the best way I knew how. I prayed a lot, talked to friends and medical staff, and tried to carry on my life as if this were just a momentary interruption, albeit a scary one.

My husband was very supportive. He made meals, kept up the housework as well as he could (cleaning and tidying up are not his forté) and took our daughter to her activities. The one thing we never did was have a serious discussion about his feelings. Was he scared for me? Not really. He always believed I would fully recover; he never once thought I would die. He was concerned for me but not overwhelmed with fear. This undoubtedly had a lot to do with my excellent prognosis.

I remember the night we took our son out for his birthday dinner. Peter was a college student, living on campus in our hometown. We told him I was going to have a breast biopsy that week but that there was really nothing to worry about since most lumps are benign. That was pretty much the extent of the conversation. Then we ate our dinner. When the lump turned out to be malignant, we told him the details of what was to be done but always focused on the positive outcome we hoped for. It wasn't until our son was engaged that I found out through his fiancée that he was very worried about me. Again, we had no serious heart-to-heart conversations. Our method of handling it was on a day-to-day basis. As my story indicated, I did very well so we just never discussed it further.

Our daughter was ten years old so we gave her the same basic explanation that we had given our son. We never emphasized the negative possibilities for her or our son, nor did we have discussions about what could happen if my medical report were really bad. We did periodically ask her how she was doing, but we never noticed any adverse effect on her.

You could say we operated by a tell-and-watch method: tell the basics and watch for problems. Maybe that was naive on our part, but we had never had lessons in cancer. We did our best.

Each family has its own style of handling crises. Whether talking out every detail or sharing only major decisions is your style, I would say do what feels right for your family. If talking about your emotions makes you feel better, then by all means discuss what is on your heart. If you are a more private person, that's okay too. But if you get stuck, depressed, or are facing communication roadblocks, seek professional help. Otherwise, allow yourself the confidence that the way you are handling your diagnosis of cancer is unique to you and it need not be compared to other ways. You have enough to be concerned about without feeling guilty about your approach to cancer.

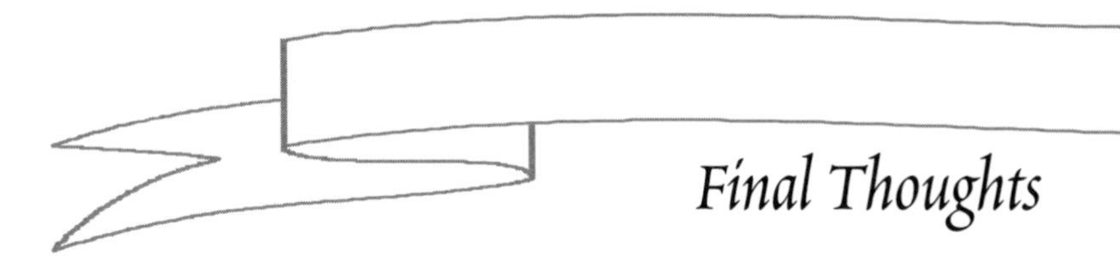

Final Thoughts

I hope my story and the added accounts of these eight women has helped you to clearly understand God's love and faithfulness. None of us were ever alone. None of us were abandoned to a life without the caring touch, prayer, or loving gesture of a person carefully chosen by God. Our needs were met and our lives became more precious because of our suffering. In turn, we have learned to help others. As the Apostle Paul tells us in II Corinthians 1:3-4, God's compassion has comforted us so we can in turn comfort others.

My prayer is that you, too, will come to trust and rely on God's love, especially during difficult times. His love is genuine. Call on Him anytime. May you have a sense of peace as you realize you are never alone. God is with you, every step of the way.

Finally, I want to leave you with some practical things you can do if you or a loved one face cancer or any serious illness. I have included some Guidelines for Prayer; Suggestions for Family, Friends and Caregivers; and Suggestions for the Person in Crisis. In addition, I have included the favorite Bible verses of the women I interviewed in the hopes that you find comfort in God's Word as well.

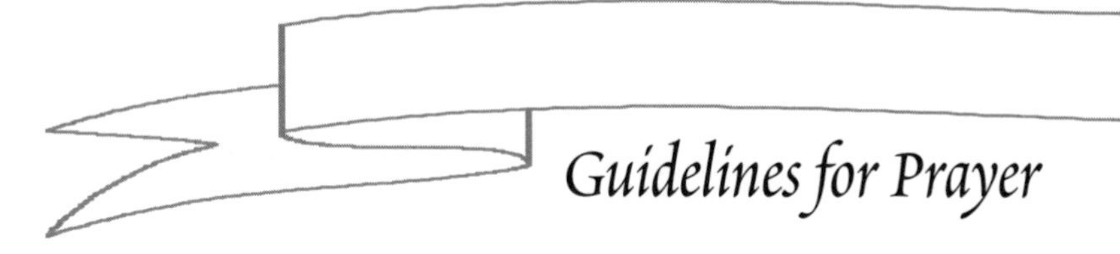

Guidelines for Prayer

Simply stated, prayer is a conversation with God. If you can talk to your spouse, your family, your friends, you can talk to God. He is an excellent listener and He would love to hear from you, especially now that you are in crisis.

> *I just pray to the Lord like He's my friend. I tell Him when I'm in a lot of pain and ask Him to relieve it.*
>
> **Elaine**

1. Talk to God.

Think of God as your Father or your very best friend. Tell Him all your concerns, your needs and your joys and sorrows in your own language. Have an on-going conversation with Him any time of the day. You can talk during your commute to work, during your walk, before bed, when you wake up, in the shower, as you clean the house and in the doctor's office. Try asking God questions. What does He want to say to you today? What can He tell you about your current situation? God would love to hear from you anywhere and any time.

One thing to keep in mind—if words won't come, a simple, "Help!" or "Be with me," is all you need to say.

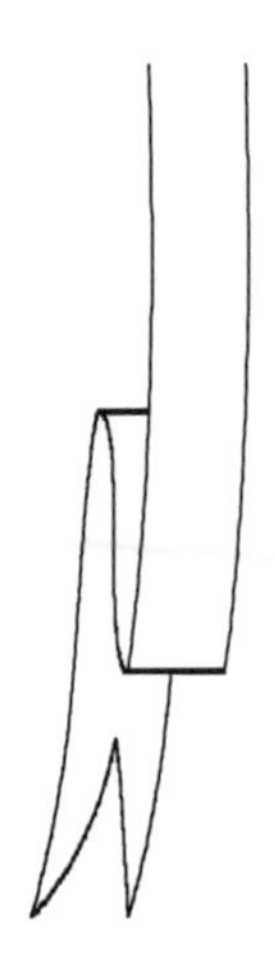

In the same way,
the Spirit helps us in our weakness.

We do not know what we ought to pray for,
but the Spirit Himself intercedes for us
with groans that words cannot express.

ROMANS 8:26

2. ***Tell Him your fears and then ask for peace of mind.***
   Are you afraid of test results, chemotherapy reactions, pain, surgery, telling your family? Are you afraid of being alone? Whatever the fear, tell God the specifics and ask him to address your fears and bring you peace about your situation. Remember Sherry's story? When she told God how afraid she was in the hospital, He sent a nurse to take her hand and comfort her. She called this "God's instant answer to prayer." God will answer your prayers, too.

3. ***Pray for competent medical staff: doctors, nurses, lab technicians, anesthesiologist.***
   God knows these people and wants you to have the very best care. Pray for skill, alertness, attention to detail, a keen

awareness of your particular diagnosis, and above all, sensitivity in how they talk to you.

4. *Ask God to heal you.*

As I explained in the beginning of my book, three of the women whom I interviewed have died of breast cancer. Sherry, Elaine, and Glenda were praying, faithful, God-fearing women and yet they died. Not all people are healed. I cannot answer the "why."

Again, what I can tell you is that God carried these women through to the end. He showed mercy by sending soft touches and gentle words of comfort, sometimes from total strangers. I believe physical healing is secondary. God's love is primary, always there, in countless ways: a kind deed, a friend's offer to pray, a meal from a neighbor, a visit from a friend.

As you ask God to heal you, focus on continuing and deepening your relationship with Him. Study Jesus' words and the healings He performed. Remember that our physical bodies are not eternal, but our spirit and character do have eternal significance. Even if we don't understand suffering and disease, we can still be secure in God's goodness and love.

5. *Tell God your feelings.*

Are you angry with God, your family, the universe, yourself? Tell Him and then ask Him to help you deal with your anger. Maybe you need to go for a long walk, call a friend, confide in your spouse. Perhaps you need some professional counseling. Don't carry this anger alone.

6. ***Listen to God.***
   He speaks to us in many ways: through the Bible, through friends and family, through nature, through the church. Listen carefully and take advantage of His wisdom.

7. ***Select your prayer partner wisely.***
   It's a good idea to have a prayer partner, someone who can be relied on for support and comfort throughout your journey. But a word of caution: avoid people who try to "fix" you with their advice, or those who tell you horror stories about someone who had the same diagnosis as yours and is now either struggling terribly with treatment or is dead. You don't need people who feed your fears. Ask God to provide you with a prayer partner who will be good for you. This may not be someone you know well, nor someone you particularly like. Actually, someone who is less personally involved in your life is probably better. God can use anyone to help you.

   My closest friend and I have prayed together over a period of time. The fact that we can call each other for prayer, about all kinds of things, has been very helpful.

   Janet

Note: I want to thank Mary Ellen Conners who helped me talk through these guidelines for prayer as well as the following suggestions.

Suggestions for Family, Friends and Caregivers

1. ***Pray for and with the person in crisis.***
   Try praying on the phone if you can't be there in person. A simple prayer can greatly reduce anxiety. Ask for specific prayer requests. Healing may not be their first priority. Freedom from fear, family issues, or a particular child's reaction may be more on their mind.

2. ***Pray for the spouse.***
   This is best done privately so that true feelings can be shared without fear of falling apart in front of their loved one.

   In many ways, cancer is harder on the spouse. He or she can be overcome with the burdens of managing the household chores, the children's activities, the laundry and the bills. There may be a feeling of helplessness and fear. What happens if their loved one dies? Then there is the guilt for having these concerns in the first place. How could their added responsibilities be worth discussing when their main focus should be caregiving.

   Pray that the spouse will find a place of support and prayer with people who can understand and share these burdens.

Perhaps you could be that support or you know someone who could. Don't let them become isolated. They need others to confirm their sanity during this difficult period and to tell them that their thoughts and feelings are normal.

3. ***Offer to help before you are asked.***
   Perhaps you could run a few errands, baby-sit while the person gets treatment, drive to appointments, water plants, walk the dog, or drive children to activities.

4. ***Hug and warmly touch.***
   There is nothing like a physical demonstration of your care. Remember, cancer is not contagious.

5. ***Listen to concerns.***
   Sometimes the best gift you can give is an open heart, open ears and a closed mouth. They are not looking for you to give them pat answers or worldly wisdom. They need you just to be there and to listen. Let them talk out whatever is on their heart. Resist the urge to offer advice.

6. ***Create diversions.***
   Think of fun things to do together, being mindful of any limitations. You could visit the zoo, the arboretum, an art gallery, go for a drive in the country, or find a new place for lunch.

7. *Laugh and cry together.*

Laughter really is great for the soul. Rent some funny movies, watch children at play, or play funny games. Then, if the mood changes, be willing to accept tears. Be vulnerable and open to sharing sadness.

8. *Give flowers or another small gift.*

Flowers in the middle of winter are a witness to the promise of spring. One flower can say it all. Smooth, silky lotion can also be a good gift.

I think one of the most helpful gifts I received was lotion. It was a bottle of creamy, pleasant smelling body lotion which helped me get used to body changes following surgery.

Lois

9. *Provide meals or other special food gifts.*

Make meals, bring an ice cream treat or some cheese and a loaf of homemade bread. Even if the person in crisis is capable of cooking, a homemade meal or any gift of food is always appreciated, especially by the person who now has cooking responsibilities.

Suggestions for the Person in Crisis

1. *Pray, particularly for your spouse and loved ones.*

In addition to the Guidelines on the previous pages, pray for sensitivity to your spouse's way of handling the details of your changed circumstances. If you have always been the cook in the family, don't criticize when your favorite dish is made with canned green beans instead of the fresh ones you would have used. And when the towels aren't folded your way, try to smile and say, "Thank you for all you do to care for me."

Remember, your spouse and loved ones may be more worried than they are letting on. Talk to them about their concerns and try to comfort them as much as you are able. Pray for their strength and peace of mind. Without making them feel guilty for leaving you, suggest that they spend some time away from you with friends or alone. Give them time to get renewed. Recognize their need to recharge.

2. *Ask for help when you need it.*

Now is the time to accept help from family and friends who will be more than willing to assist you in any number of ways. Try to give them specific things to do and then lean back and relax. You can reciprocate in the future.

3. ***Journal.***
   If you've never tried journaling, now is the time. Write down everything that is happening to you and your family and be sure to include your feelings. Then ask God what He has to say to you. Turn off your brain and listen to God. Record the thoughts that come. God will show up and guide you through difficult times.

4. ***Celebrate milestones.***
   I read about one woman who bought a plain straw hat. At the completion of each treatment, she attached a new silk flower to the brim. Now she has a beautiful flowered hat as a permanent reminder of her journey. Why not celebrate a good white cell count, the selection of the perfect wig, or a negative test result?

5. ***Say "I love you" more often.***
   When was the last time you told your spouse, your children, your parents and your friends that you love them? Life is short. Tell them now.

6. ***Settle disputes and if possible, reconcile.***
   If it is at all within your control, settle old wounds. Learn to forgive so you can let go of bitterness and enjoy life fully.

7. ***Eat healthy foods and exercise as directed by your doctor.***
   Talk to your doctor and a good dietitian about anti-oxidant foods and appropriate exercise following surgery. Don't be

afraid to ask for a referral to a physical therapist to get back in shape.

8. ***Pay attention to your emotions.***
   - Lighten up and laugh.

   Rent a funny movie, read humorous books, call up friends who make you laugh, find humor in everyday life.

   - Cry when you need to.

   There will be times when you'll need to cry. Let the tears flow freely. If you think you are having a problem with depression, seek medical attention.

9. ***Do things that will feed your spirit.***
   Listen to praise music; read a favorite Psalm morning and night or have someone else read it to you or listen to a tape of healing Scriptures. Surround yourself with a community of faith who will lift you up when you are down.

10. ***Remember that God can still use you in the midst of your illness.***
    Ask God to fill you with the fruit of the Spirit found in Galations 5:22: "love, joy, peace, patience, kindness, goodness, faithfulness, gentleness and self-control." You can be a powerful witness to God's love during this time and you may unknowingly lead people to a relationship with Christ. In our weakness, God is strong!

God is in control of everything. He is sovereign and I trust Him. My illness will be used for His glory. Regardless of what happens to me physically, I want the Lord to be honored and for this to touch lives.

Janet

Helpful Bible Verses

I asked the Lord to give me a verse of Scripture that I could hold onto. The Scripture I got was: "*For I know the plans I have for you,*" *declares the Lord,* "*plans to prosper you and not to harm you, plans to give you hope and a future.*" (Jeremiah 29:11)

And it was like all the time the Lord was saying, "*So do not fear, for I am with you…*" (Isaiah 41:10)

Elaine

When all this started, early on my oldest daughter, who was 15 at the time, got on the computer and printed Jeremiah 29:11. And I still have it on my refrigerator to this day: "*Plans for good and not for evil.*" (paraphrased) I think that would probably be THE one most meaningful verse for me. Just because she printed that for me and it's there in front of me everyday. And because that does give you hope.

Julia

Could there be anything better than God's peace which passes all understanding? *And the peace of God, which transcends all understanding, will guard your hearts and your minds in Christ Jesus*. (Philippians 4:7)

Lois

I like James 1:2 because it talks about trials: *Consider it pure joy, my brothers, whenever you face trials of many kinds...* Another one talks about trial—because I really thought it was a trial. *In this you greatly rejoice, though now for a little while you may have had to suffer grief in all kinds of trials*. (I Peter 1:6) So I keep thinking there is a reason for us to have a trial and the outcome has to be left to God.

Nini

I found this Bible verse when we were doing our Bible study: ...*And I pray that you, being rooted and established in love, may have power, together with all the saints, to grasp how wide and long and high and deep is the love of Christ*. (Ephesians 3:17) And it just really, really spoke to me about how when we're rooted in Christ then He shows us how wide and long and high and deep His love is and that we're filled to the measure with the fullness of God. And that He can do more than we ask or imagine, according to His power. And I think it boils down to we can do what we think is best and we can go to these clinics and have treatments, and all of that is fine. It's been proven to be helpful. But Christ is the one with the power and honor. He knows the future. We just have to cling to Him. I don't know how people survive and thrive who don't have faith. I really don't.

Kory

Joshua 1:9 was my lifeline. *"Have I not commanded you? Be strong and courageous. Do not be terrified; do not be discouraged, for the Lord your God will be with you wherever you go."* That verse is on the quilt that my niece made for me. It's covered with the healing hands of my family and friends. Healing hands. It's a pretty neat quilt.

Sherry

I meditated on Matthew 16:15—*"But what about you?"* He *asked. "Who do you say I am?"* Now that's a good verse. Look at the attributes of God, His character. If I really believe what God's character is and embrace it in my heart, my life will change. He is the King of the universe. Trust Him for everything. Call on Him regarding everything. Depend totally on Him because He is all sufficient.

Janet

I like: *Love is patient, love is kind. It does not envy, it does not boast, it is not proud.* (I Corinthians 13:4)

Glenda

And the peace of God, which transcends all understanding, will guard your hearts and your minds in Christ Jesus. (Philippians 4:7)

Pam

Every Step of the Way

A Faith Journey Through Breast Cancer

Order Form

Need another copy for a friend or support group? You can order directly from:

Pam Lillehei
P.O. Box 240584
Apple Valley, MN 55124
Phone: (952) 431-0721
e-mail: PamLillehei@aol.com

Number of Copies	________ x	$14.95	________
Tax (MN residents only)	Plus 6.5%		________
Shipping—one book		$ 2.95	________
Shipping—additional copies	________ x	$ 1.00	________
	TOTAL ORDER		________

Payment Enclosed: Check or Money Order

Shipping Address

Name (please print) ________________________________

Address ________________________________

City ____________________ *State* ______ *Zip* __________

Telephone (_____) ____________________________